Ooh La La!

ALSO BY JAMIE CAT CALLAN

French Women Don't Sleep Alone

Bonjour, Happiness!

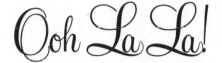

Ooh La La!

FRENCH WOMEN'S SECRETS TO FEELING BEAUTIFUL EVERY DAY

JAMIE CAT CALLAN

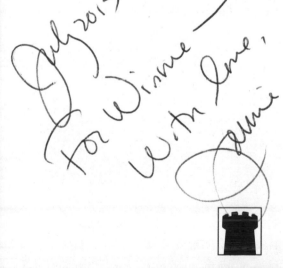

CITADEL PRESS
Kensington Publishing Corp.
www.kensingtonbooks.com

CITADEL PRESS BOOKS are published by

Kensington Publishing Corp.
119 West 40th Street
New York, NY 10018

All Kensington titles, imprints, and distributed lines are available at special quantity discounts for bulk purchases for sales promotions, premiums, fund-raising, educational, or institutional use. Special book excerpts or customized printings can also be created to fit specific needs. For details, write or phone the office of the Kensington special sales manager: Kensington Publishing Corp., 119 West 40th Street, New York, NY 10018, attn: Special Sales Department; phone 1-800-221-2647.

CITADEL PRESS and the Citadel logo are Reg. U.S. Pat. & TM Off.

First printing: June 2013

10 9 8 7 6 5 4 3 2 1

Printed in the United States of America

CIP data is available.

ISBN-13: 978-0-8065-3557-9
ISBN-10: 0-8065-3557-1

First electronic edition: June 2013

ISBN-13: 978-0-8065-3558-6
ISBN-10: 0-8065-3558-X

For Marceline

Let us leave pretty women to men with no imagination.
—MARCEL PROUST

Contents

Prologue

A FUNNY THING happened on the way to writing this book.

Well, actually, maybe not so funny. But certainly, *interesting*.

One lovely autumn evening, as I was stepping out to have dinner with friends in Toulouse, I encountered a very large cobblestone. The pointed toe of my shoe got caught underneath it, and with my foot trapped there, I slipped and twisted my ankle, this way and then that. And just as an aside—I was not wearing high heels. The pain was so intense I immediately passed out. When I came to, my friends were kneeling beside me and I could hear the sounds of the French ambulance careening down the narrow street to fetch me. I was lifted onto a stretcher and rushed to the local hospital, where I ended up staying for nine days at which point my husband who had been in Australia on a scientific research trip came to France to get me and bring me home. As it turns out I had broken my ankle in two different places and I needed major surgery. I am now the proud owner of an ankle that contains a metal plate and six screws inserted into it.

So you see, when I do something, I don't do it halfway.

With all those hours lying in bed—much of it spent on morphine—I had plenty of time to contemplate the secrets of French women.

I had spent the previous month traveling around France, interviewing French women—some close friends, some ac-

1

quaintances, and some whom I had just met for the specific purpose of writing this book; by the time I ended up in the hospital, I still had not yet quite cracked the code on the secret to a French woman's allure. I had all the pieces, but I still had not quite put the puzzle together. Something was still missing.

And so, lying there in the hospital bed, my left leg hoisted up, staring out the window at the blue-blue skies of Toulouse, pondering the clouds, I began to dream about my French grandmother. As a child, I often spent my summers with her. We would sit on her porch, drinking her lemony iced tea while my grandfather worked in the garden. And in the late afternoons, she insisted I take a nap. I still remember lying down on the living room sofa with a couple of pillows behind my head while my grandmother would wordlessly lower the shades, blocking out the noonday sun, throwing a soft shadow across the room. She would whisper that I should try to sleep, and then she would leave. I had no choice but to stay still and stare up at the little framed picture on the wall in front of me. Even today, this picture looms large in my memory. Perhaps you've seen it. It's a print called *Le Moulin Rouge* from an oil painting by the artist Guy Dessapt. In the picture, it's a snowy evening on the streets of Paris. Today, Parisians still sell this print to the tourists strolling along the Seine's Left Bank. But to me, as a child, it was quite special. I remember lying there, trying to stay awake, while I focused on all the details. There's the famous red windmill outside the dance hall and a sign announcing MOULIN ROUGE in lights. As my eyes became heavy and just before wandering off to dreamland, I began to imagine what happened inside that theater. Certainly, there would be dancing. Pretty women, of course. Feathers. Sequins. Bright lights. Oh, and music! A spectacular show every night of the week. I should mention here that my grandparents and my mother and uncle were in a Vaudeville troupe during the Great Depression. Perhaps this is why the picture of the Moulin Rouge captivated me so much. In fact, after a month in France, I came to believe that this picture was an important clue when it came to discovering my own *ooh la la.*

Now, I'm not saying that you're going to find your *ooh la la* staring at a picture of the Moulin Rouge or even from a trip to France. You might find your *ooh la la* on a farm in Kansas or while playing the piano, or a game of tennis. Then again, your *ooh la la* might be waiting for you in a ship out at sea or in the middle of downtown Chicago or in a classroom in Japan. Maybe your *ooh la la* is in a garden or at a library.

For me, at age fifty-eight with a grown-up daughter and newly remarried, I did discover my *ooh la la* in France, but it took some effort and perhaps even breaking my ankle to truly see that it had been standing right in front of me all along.

It took gallivanting around Paris, traveling to the north of France as far up as the Belgian border, through parts of Normandy, spending time in the city of Rouen where Joan of Arc spent her final days, and then through the south to the little village of Auvillar and the big city of Toulouse—all in an effort to discover why French women have this reputation for being so mysterious and sexy and beautiful and confident.

I learned about perfume, skin care, style, fashion, lingerie, and makeup.

However, I also learned about a lot of things that simply cannot be distilled into little beauty tips; for example, *always spritz your face in the evening with Evian*. (Although one French friend of mine swears by this, and she does have lovely skin!)

Rather, after all these interviews and meetings, I began to realize that there is something deeper to the French woman's beauty and elegance and mystery. And this something goes beyond fashion tips and beauty makeovers. So yes, while I learned some great ideas about how to keep your skin glowing, choose a signature fragrance and how to find the perfect accent color for you (all included in this book), I also learned about something deeper and much more elusive. And something beyond mere physical beauty. I like to call it *ooh la la*.

We've all heard this expression *ooh la la*! It originated in France in the 1920s and now many Americans have adopted it as a way of saying that something is chic or sexy or fun or just plain wonderful. And while I started off writing a book about French beauty, I soon realized that the real reason many of us find French women so captivating and fascinating is not merely because they are beautiful, but because of something deeper.

Through all my research and note taking, I came to realize that the French woman's true allure comes from the fact that she obviously feels total permission to be completely herself. Still, this is not something you can find in a bottle or in a cream or at a sample sale. It's not something you can get from an injection or from a filler or even from a lift. It's something that you cultivate and develop during a lifetime. It involves patience and courage and love and lots of imagination. Ah, but here's the great news about *ooh la la*—it's available to any woman (whether you live in Boston or Brazil, whether you're rich or poor, whether you've traveled the world or never left your own backyard). In fact, it's available to any woman who wants to break away from the pack and be her own unique beautiful self.

Once you read this book, it is my hope that you will begin your own search for *ooh la la*, and that the stories here will help inspire you on your particular journey. It is my aim that the French women's secrets I've revealed here will open doors inside your own heart, so that you may find the courage and the love to be your most authentic self—your best self. Your happiest, wisest, sexiest, and most beautiful and generous self.

!!!

CHAPTER ONE

You Had Me at Bonjour

How many cares one loses when one decides not to be
something, but to be someone.

—COCO CHANEL

IT IS A WARM September day and I am in Paris, waiting in the
reception area for my friend Isabelle. Isabelle is only in her
late twenties, but this gal is wise beyond her years.

I sit on a little couch with a good view of the elevators
and stairs, so I get to observe the French men and women,
coming and going. Even from this very superficial viewpoint,
it's obvious that French professionals—or at least Parisian
professionals—dress up more than Americans do. There doesn't
seem to be a *casual Friday*, which has turned into a *casual
all-week-long*. Still, I will say this, there are women wearing
jeans, but they are stylish and well tailored, and the women
add a cute blazer, a silk blouse, and always a scarf. Mostly, I
see lots of skirts paired with boots. The skirts graze the knees
so you catch just a glimpse of textured stockings. It's pretty,
elegant, and intriguing.

Before long, Isabelle arrives. I stand to greet her, and in

one simple sweep, she gently touches my shoulder and turns her head quickly this way, and then that, for the *bises*. The French greeting—the kiss on each cheek. *Hello, Jamie!* she says happily. She pronounces my name *Jeemmee* and it sounds so pretty, dressed up in this French accent, that I don't have the heart to correct her. She loves practicing her English with me and so for now, I am *Jeemmee*.

As we gather our things, I notice that Isabelle looks very different from the last time I saw her. She's cut her hair shorter and she now has gold highlights. On our Métro ride to her condo outside Paris in Boulogne-Billancourt, Isabelle tells me all about Madame Josie Mermet. Isabelle recently had a "re-imaging" session with her at the department store Printemps, and she tells me that Josie has changed her life!

It's true—since I last stayed with Isabelle, she has indeed been truly transformed. Yes, her hair is shorter and the highlights are beautiful, but more than this, Isabelle is happier. *It's not just superficial color-analysis,* Isabelle tells me as we walk into her apartment.

Isabelle brings out a little pot of herbal tea and a plate of what she calls biscuits, and continues, *Josie Mermet reads your soul. She understands who you are meant to be in this world. It's very deep!* Isabelle hands me the little cup and saucer and turns to me. *Oh, and she's old, so she's got all that experience.* This statement I find particularly delicious. I am about twenty-five years older than Isabelle and suddenly feel so appreciated. It's not simply that this French woman is teaching me things, but I suppose I can teach her things. Even if I am American! After all, I have *experience!*

Isabelle puts her teacup down and continues. *She told me I must mix the styles up so my personality shows. And she says I have a pretty face and I need to show it. She does chromopsychology. Jeemmee, you have to meet her!*

Isabelle goes to her desk and takes out a folder with lots of paper and drawings. While she does this, I bite into the biscuit and realize it's not a biscuit or a cookie. It's a cracker. Hmm . . . it's not sweet, but it's tasty.

This is my chromopsychology, Isabelle says, sitting down next to me and showing me a drawing and color swatches. *The stylist told me I need to wear more earth tones. Rust colors, warm browns, and golds.* Isabelle glides her hand through her silky brunette hair. *See?* And I do—it's lovely and the tone does bring out her eyes.

As I look around Isabelle's apartment, I see how all this makes sense. She has lots of posters of wolves (she tells me she loves wolves), but also there's an Indian print bedspread pinned to one wall and a poster of dolphins swimming with the words LIVE FREE in English and another poster with a photograph of a beach and palm trees in the orange light of sunset. The apartment's décor is awash in browns and golds and deep greens. Clearly, she's a gal who loves nature and the great outdoors.

I look at the drawings from her chromopsychology session. Each one features a line drawing of a heart-shaped-face woman. There are colors applied to her lips, cheeks, and eyes, and little notes on the side with names of specific colors and products. At first glance, I think this is a typical beauty makeover with color analysis, but I see that it is so much more. Josie Mermet sketches out clothing styles, haircut, and color, accessories that not only compliment a woman's skin or body type, but also her personality. She bases her recommendations on the woman's background, her childhood, her preoccupations, and her dreams for the future. Isabelle tells me that there are thirty types and that she is a "granite." Josie told her that she likes to help others. Certainly, that's true, I think as she pours us more tea. Outside the sun is setting.

I'm Aries with Libra rising, Isabelle says, showing me lists of makeup, types of handbags that will suit her personality, bijoux, belts, shoes, scarves, handbags. And then there's a list, "Ten Things You Should Have in Your Wardrobe," with the suggestion that Isabelle should dress more romantically and combine leather with softer, more flowing fabrics. And again, I can see how this will be perfect for her.

Isabelle turns to me and says with great passion, *Jeemmee, you must meet Josie Mermet. She will help you with your book.* And I agree. I must meet this Madame Josie Mermet and I must learn all about this chromopsychology business!

And so, phone calls are made and appointments confirmed. I am going to meet Josie at her office on the Right Bank, not far from the famous department store Printemps.

But first I must get to the appointment, which is not easy, because I must make several switches on the Métro—going from the dark yellow line on the Left Bank to the light purple line to Invalides and then getting off there and switching to the bright green line, which takes me to Haussman Saint-Lazare on the Right Bank. I'm being very specific about the colors because there are three different shades of green, and the route depends on the color of the Métro line, plus what direction you're going in. Oh, and the routes have numbers, too! Truthfully, it's all very circuitous, this French Métro system, and I always feel as if my brain is getting a great workout—a wordless exercise in following routes that begin and then split up and then split again, with me dashing around and around through the brightly tiled corridors, feeling a little bit like I'm inside a pinball machine, spinning around and around. And then after much stair climbing up and down, with colorful billboards advertising perfumes and plays and the latest collection at Galleries Lafayette, and going around and around some more, I am finally spit out at my destination. Still, I confess—I love riding the Métro!

And now, here I am on this perfectly sunny day, standing in front of the window of a Francis L. Rhod, Haute Coiffure Française on rue Taitbout, staring at my own reflection into a hair salon. The girls in the salon stare back at me as if to say *who is this American standing outside the salon staring at us through the window?* I check my little notebook. Yes, I have the correct address. And then I see in the corner of the window, a little sign that Josie Mermet does her re-imaging consultations here. I am in the right place after all, and so I enter the salon and tell the receptionist that I am here to interview Madame Mermet. She asks me to wait on a white leather sofa. She offers me a glass of mineral water. I accept it. After about ten minutes, another woman approaches me, speaking softly in English with a heavy French accent. She tells me she is Celine, Madame Mermet's assistant, and that she will now bring me to meet Madame. This assistant, Celine, is really gorgeous. She has very short-cropped platinum blond hair with dark roots. It's all very cool, but very subtle. She wears a shimmery steel-gray knee-length dress that skims her slender frame. But what I really notice are her shoes—silver laced-up oxfords. And then I see she's wearing silver bangles, and even though her hair is blond, it's got this silvery tint to it and I feel as if this girl might suddenly grab my hand and insist I dance the Charleston with her.

But rather than dancing, I quickly follow her down a spiral staircase. There is always a spiral staircase in France. No matter where you go, at some point in your day, you will be walking up or down a spiral staircase. Celine smiles and says something to me about waiting there—all I hear is *attendez*—and then she is gone, disappearing behind a black velvety curtain. And then, I am seated on another white leather sofa and asked to wait.

Just as I am wondering about what's behind those curtains, they open to reveal—Madame Mermet. She is a tiny woman, dressed all in black—black straight jeans, a black top, a black jacket—it's all a bit androgynous, but very sleek and tailored. And her hair—it is jet black and cropped in this very short stylish bob. But what really gets me is her bright red-lipsticked mouth, which is very full and get this—outlined in black lipliner. Yes, her look is a bit startling, but you know what—it's also fantastic!

I catch my breath and stand up to greet her. She kisses me on each cheek and speaks so very softly, so sweetly, that for a moment I am reminded of Michael Jackson.

This thought doesn't have time to penetrate my brain, because Celine is holding the curtain open for us, waiting for me to come inside. I follow the two women into a small room with three red Louis XIV–style chairs arranged in a little circle. I sit down between Josie and Celine. I try to resist staring at Josie, but it's not easy. She has an incredibly dramatic look—yes, there's the red-lipsticked mouth, outlined in black, but also she has gorgeous hazel eyes, outlined in black kohl, and her eyebrows are a force in and of themselves. She has a beauty mark beneath her right eye. Honestly, I cannot take my eyes off her. For such a tiny woman, she has an incredibly commanding presence.

Nonetheless, I compose myself, get out my little moleskin notebook, and flip open to a blank page. I begin asking questions. Lots of questions.

Madame Mermet tells me that she began her *re-looking* work thirty years ago. For a time, she worked exclusively with L'Oreal and traveled all over the world for them, doing makeovers. She took this knowledge and experience and combined it with morphopsychology, which is the study of personality based on body type. From here, she created her own specialty, which she calls *chromopsychology*.

Here's how it works—at first, Madame Mermet just looks at the woman who's come into the office for a makeover. The client is not allowed to talk or ask questions. She is asked to stand, walk, stand again, and sit. Madame simply observes the woman's bone structure, her hair texture, her complexion, as well as her morphopsychology—her body shape, her way of walking in and out of the room, and how she presents herself. I ask Madame why her clients are not allowed to ask questions, and she responds as if this is obvious. *I work intuitively,* she says, *I make you more you.* And then, she explains that her work is based on the woman's true personality, and truly seeing this authentic self is crucial to understanding the colors, shapes, and textures that will make her shine. And this includes not just your clothing, hair, and makeup, but your home and office space, along with your jewelry and your eyeglasses. *Even the color of your car is important,* she pronounces. *The right color can give you a different spirit!*

I ask Madame Mermet about her childhood and how her passion for helping women find their truest selves began, and she tells me that she grew up in Chaumergy, a little village in Franche-Comté. As a little girl, Madame Mermet noticed that her two older sisters who were just one year apart looked so different from her. One had copper-colored hair and another was a blonde. And even her mother, she explains to me, had a different sensibility. But as a little girl, Josie who was petite and dark had to wear the hand-me-down dresses from her taller, blonder sisters, which meant wearing clothes that did not suit her at all. As she grew into her teen years, she became more aware of the differences. She experimented with a variety of looks by going through the fashion magazines and cutting up the pictures to create her own paper dolls. She would take one model and switch her face with another model's face and do the same with their bodies, clothing, shoes, bags, and accessories, rearranging all these elements to find the perfect, most pleasing, and natural sensibility.

I take notes and Madame Mermet begins talking very quickly. Celine must help with translating. Celine has been with her for over eighteen years and has the highest respect for this amazing woman. I must admit, I, too, am falling under her spell. The truth is, I would like to get her advice on what I should do—even to walk out the door understanding what type I am would be thrilling. I know I'm not a "granite," like Isabelle. She told me that Madame Mermet is a "dramatique," and I know I'm probably not that type. Well, actually, maybe I'm a little "dramatique," but certainly not in the style of Madame Mermet. And in this moment, I am feeling very American, and of all the thirty different types, I wonder if there's a type for me. I have this sinking feeling that perhaps I am no type at all.

And then, suddenly—as if reading my mind—Madame Mermet pronounces: *We respect the differences!*

She is looking directly into my eyes.. Honestly, I feel as if she is reading my mind and so I have to ask—what about body issues? Really, meaning, what if a woman is not slender? *What do you say to women about diet and exercise?* I ask. *Is that part of chromopsychology?*

And she tells me that with chromopsychology they do not talk about weight, but often a woman who needs to lose a few kilos will lose them without much effort because after her makeover, she receives so many compliments and she is in alignment with her true self, she is simply inspired to be as healthy and beautiful as possible.

But what if she has some obvious flaw? I continue. *And she's not what our world considers beautiful?* And here is where Madame Mermet gets very passionate. Her eyes grow wide and fiery and they actually seem to change from goldish-brown to green. She straightens her back, which is amazing because her posture is already impeccable, but suddenly this diminutive woman grows taller and for a fraction of a second, I see Madame Mermet as a little girl in the country, holding her head high as she suffered the indignity of being made to wear her blond sisters' pink-and-pastel-colored hand-me-downs.

We transfer the handicap and make it an asset! she tells me. And then she waves a tiny hand in the air and tells me, *we fight against the beauty norm! It kills originality and beauty!*

I confess I am flustered for a moment. This is not what I am after, really. I want to hear the French secrets to beauty. I want a list of the top ten magical beauty tricks that will be the key to opening the door to all that French *je ne sais quoi,* and this is when she declares—*There is not one standard of beauty!* And I honestly feel as if she is looking straight into my heart.

By the time I pack up my little notebook and gather up my purse and camera, bid my farewells and walk up that spiral staircase once again, I leave with the distinct feeling that I have just begun a very long, but wonderful journey in which I will be changed forever.

When you're in the presence of someone who truly knows exactly who they are in this world—it's completely thrilling. I've often felt this when I meet an excellent actress. I belonged to a theater workshop years ago, and while I was there to write plays, a director came up to me as the evening was ending and we were all going home. She stopped me and gave me the once-over. She mistook me for an actress and immediately launched into advice on what roles I should go out for. *You're not the star,* she said, scrutinizing my face, my body, my hair, my clothes, even my cute red ballet flats. *No, you're the quirky next-door neighbor. You're the funny one.* Now, this might sound like some kind of insult, but the moment the director said this, I felt the basic truth in it. I *am* the quirky next-door neighbor. I don't even want to be the perfectly beautiful star. That just doesn't sound like all that much fun, anyway, if you want to know the truth.

Now, I have no intention of getting a job on a television sitcom, but I wonder if this director's way of looking at a woman is not completely dissimilar to what Madame Josie Mermet does. I wonder if we could help ourselves by looking in the mirror as if we were a director and asking ourselves—what role should that woman in the mirror play? Is she dark and brooding? Sweet and funny? Brilliant and complicated? Where would you place her? In the mountains, hiking? In a pool in Los Angeles? On a desert island? In a big city? And what would we tell the costume department? Oh, and while we're at it—is she in a contemporary scene or should she be placed in the 1920s wearing a fringed flapper dress?

I know that this line of questioning can't replace a trip to Paris and a session with the brilliant Josie Mermet, but I do think it's a beginning.

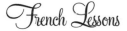

Find a mentor. This may be easier in a service-oriented society such as France, but it's still possible in America. True, in America we tend to be rugged individualists and so we're more of a self-service society. I know for myself, I don't always trust salesladies, and I have more than a few friends who feel the same way. (Although, I make an exception with Nordstrom's—those gals are very helpful!) Still, I think we're a little suspicious of salespeople who want to help us pick out something as simple as a new lipstick. I think this is because we worry that they're just trying to sell us something—anything—and they don't really care about getting to know what's right for us (which is another way of saying what's special about us) because well— that salesgirl or waiter or beauty adviser is not in it for the long run. While they're describing the benefits of some new skincare product, they are really thinking about how they'll skip out by five o'clock so they can make it to the audition for America's Next Top Model. And once their Hollywood ship comes in, it's so long beauty counter!

And so, as Americans, I think we often go it alone in terms of our beauty needs. This is not the case for French women. For them, it's all about finding the right person— a mentor—someone who will guide them through the in-

tricacies of discovering their own unique look and style. Yes, French women are just like us—they read the latest fashion and beauty magazines—but it's more important for them to find that one woman—that expert mentor who can truly help them achieve the look that is uniquely right for them.

In addition to all this, the French women I interviewed are very big on things like aura cleansing, visiting psychics, and even the Tarot. Not just for their future love lives or career paths, but for beauty and style advice. I'm not suggesting we should all run out and buy a pack of Tarot cards and dabble in the occult, but here's what I think is interesting and what I learned from Josie Mermet—French women's notion of beauty starts with their psychic selves. And from there, they tune into their personalities, their uniqueness, and even the knowledge of what they are meant to do in this lifetime and who they are meant to be. Then, with this foundation, they decide whether glossy pink lipstick is going to look good on them or perhaps they should wear more crushed velvet and then again, perhaps they need to cut their hair very short and dye it jet-black and wear black skinny jeans with a red mouth outlined in black lipliner.

So, here's your French lesson—find a mentor. You can start by enlisting the help of a trusted friend, a sister, your mother or your grandmother. Find someone who "gets" you and wants only the best for you. Find a woman you can trust. Next, find a makeup artist who you can go to for advice that is specific to your personality. Find a hairdresser who understands your hair type and your unique style. Oh, and whenever you visit your hairdresser or beauty adviser or personal shopper, dress up. Be the person you want to become—even if it feels as if you are playing a role. This way, you will send out the message to the world about your truest self, and you will open the door to become the woman you were always meant to be.

Finally, look at yourself as if you were a director, casting for parts in a new movie. Now, consider what role you'd like to play on this stage called life. And then, be the star.

Or the quirky next-door neighbor, if you like!

!!!

CHAPTER TWO

~

Am I Blue?

Colors, like features, follow the changes of the emotions.

—PABLO PICASSO

MICHELINE TANGUY has asked me to meet her at her favorite café in the Marais—a historic neighborhood in Paris known for its art galleries, trendy restaurants, and chic little shops. Micheline has chosen this particular café so that we can practice the French sport of *Le Regard*, or as we Americans call it, people watching. She has promised me that together we will deconstruct the French look and uncover exactly what makes the French woman so alluring. So, I take the Métro and get off at the Hotel Ville stop.

I met Micheline a few years ago in Paris at an organized dinner party group called Paris Soirees. Patricia Laplant-Collins organizes these fabulous dinner parties, and I was asked to give a talk about my book—to mostly expats living in Paris, but there were a few French people there, and Micheline was one of them. After the talk, she hurried up to me just as I was leaving and cornered me by the coat closet. *I must talk to you!* she said quickly, smiling widely, her eyes lit up. She's a tiny thing—dark hair, dark eyes, olive skin, and that night she was dressed in a classic white blouse and black pencil skirt. Heels, of course. There was so much excitement in this little body that it seemed she would burst. *Jeemmee, I must tell you something!* She whispered this with such intensity, I admit, I was a little scared. This is because, after my first book came out, I often found myself confronted with a French woman saying, *excuse me, but I am a real French woman, and I have to tell you—I sleep alone!*

So, there!

But this is not what Micheline wanted to tell me. Rather, she wanted to talk about something much deeper. The nature of love. The secret to happiness. What it means to be a woman. I admit, this pretty woman had grabbed my attention. She's around my age, but truthfully there was so much energy and enthusiasm, I felt as if I was speaking to a much younger, very wise woman. She looked at me and said, *the secret is you are Woman!* And here she pounded her heart with her little fist. *Just be!*

I was smitten. Obviously this French woman could tell me a thing or two. And so, on my next trip to France, we agreed to meet. She would help me understand the simplicity of just "being" and how French women cultivate their confidence, their mystery, and their allure.

In America, we would probably call Micheline an image consultant; however, for her, this idea of building an image is only a part of what she does for a client, and so she is actually called a "charisma expert." I gather that this is something like an image consultant, in that she helps businesswomen and -men learn to be charming and negotiate the cultural crossroads between France and their home country.

There is clearly a lot of this cross-cultural business happening all over France. I notice tons of advertisements on the Métro that shout out —*Avez-vous la langue bien pendue?* I suspect they're talking about how well you can speak the language. The literal translation is *How well is your tongue hung?* Underneath this it says, "Learn Wall Street English," and there's a picture of a very attractive man, but more often, a pretty young woman sticking out her tongue to show it's been painted to look like the American flag. Sometimes, the attractive woman has a British flag painted on her tongue, but it seems to me the Wall Street English wins out in the popularity contest. The message is clear—if you want to do business in today's economy, you must learn to speak English. It seems to me that the French are selling this idea of speaking English in your professional life as something vaguely sexy. Or maybe not even vaguely sexy, but very sexy.

I meet Micheline at the café. She is wearing a gray-toned three-quarter-length jacket with trousers that are in the same tonal family, along with a crisp white blouse that emphasizes her tan and her dark hair.

Micheline tells me that she helps people find their charisma by teaching them the art of *savoir faire*—how to dress, move, speak, and basically how to be attractive, appropriate, and worldly. But it's the part about being attractive that most interests me. I wonder what exactly she means by teaching charisma and if this is the secret to *ooh la la.*

We settle ourselves at an outdoor table under the awning. It is a Wednesday morning around eleven and so the café is fairly empty. But the streets are still slick from an early-morning rainfall, which has just now stopped. Passersby toting shopping bags hurry past the café. We position ourselves so that the tiny table is between us and so that we have a good view of the street scene. Micheline and I order a couple of espressos, and before I know it, we are off and running with *le projet du jour.* People watching.

For a few minutes, Micheline is silent and I ask her what perfume she's wearing. *White Linen from Estée Lauder,* she tells me.

An American fragrance! I say, a little excited.

She shrugs her shoulders and says, *why not?*

Yes, indeed. Why not?

And then we return our gaze to the street. Men and women come and go, mostly it seems to me—going in one direction. Toward something. Perhaps there is an office nearby? I notice a certain crispness to them. They definitely look more elegant than their American counterparts. I try to deconstruct why. Yes, the scarves make a big difference. It's not just the fact that there's a color accent and something to coordinate with a belt or shoes or a pocketbook. It's a finishing touch, and for a woman, I think, it's similar to a man wearing a tie. Micheline tells me the scarf is for protection. Micheline pronounces the word—*pro-teck-shion*—and then gestures to her throat; I get the sense that the scarf is not simply for protection against the elements, but it is a kind of armor that will protect a woman from unknown assailants, court intrigues, and malcontents of all kinds.

Yes, my imagination is having a bit of a field day. This always happens to me when I sit at a café. More so, I believe because I am with Micheline, who tells me to look at this woman's shoes. *They are not new, you see, but they are beautiful. She takes good care of them.* And then to notice another woman's walk. *It is the good posture that makes the difference, non?* I nod my head and think about this and then quickly straighten my shoulders and elongate my neck.

It's important to be attractive at first for ourselves, she tells me. *We do our best to reach this aim in our daily life. It's not only the appearance. It's also self-esteem, confidence, and respect for ourselves.*

Suddenly, we both look up as another woman comes into view. She is wearing purple leggings and a fabulous purple and black diamond-patterned dress. Her hair is hennaed red. *Ooh la la!* I say and turn to Micheline, who has taken out a cigarette from a little blue enamel case. *Non!* She tells me.

She's not French? I ask.

Micheline lights up her cigarette and takes a moment. She is thinking. After a bit, she says, *I'm giving this up,* waving her hand at the smoke in the air. *I'm down to three cigarettes a day. It takes time.* Then she turns her head to the woman in purple. *Maybe she's French. I don't know. It's a good possibility she is French. This is not the point. Anyway, French women, they can have bad dress.*

I raise my eyes at her. Is this true? I wonder. If so, then my whole world is going to shatter. I don't know what I'll do. If I can't look to French women as my spiritual fashion guides, then what am I doing?

Micheline stubs out her cigarette. *A woman must be in alignment,* she says.

Alignment with what? I ask.

Herself! Her story about herself. So if she is French, then be French. If you are an American, be an American, but be yourself. Let your style tell your story.

Micheline goes on to explain to me that French women are uniquely aware that they do not really control their future. Things change and all one can do is take care of the present. *You can't take anything for granted,* she tells me. *It is important to work with what you have. Have a con-*

versation between your ego and your heart. This is an ongoing conversation whether we're talking about chocolate or a new dress. And I look at Micheline and realize that I don't often live in the present and that this has gotten me into some trouble in my life. I am often leaping toward the next thing and not appreciating what is right here before me. And part of this is the penchant to live on credit. French women don't have our style of credit cards, but rather something called *Carte Bleue*, which is kind of like our ATM debit cards, and there are no bank fees.

We pay the bill, and Micheline gives me a knowing glance, before we hit the streets of Marais. She walks fast, expertly weaving in and out of the crowds on the street. She points out the landmarks to me. We walk down rue des Francs-Bourgeois and look at the shops and then stroll down the historic Jewish quarter and over to the Pompidou Center and finally over to Le Hangar where we get a table in the outdoor café. From this vantage point we are able to do more people watching, plus we enjoy a really fine lunch of duck breast and then a salad (we skip the cheese course), along with a glass of wine. White for me, red for Micheline. Oh, and finally an espresso and some lemon sorbet.

After lunch, it's time for shopping! Micheline leads me through a courtyard and into a very elegant shop. She tells me that she will teach me about colors. And how they play a powerful role in a woman's wardrobe, but also in her charisma. We stop at a display table full of scarves. She picks out some plum-colored ones and holds them up to my face. I look in the mirror. I look horrible. The color absolutely drains everything from my face. It's actually scary. At first, I think Micheline does not know her colors—if she thinks that plum looks good on a blond-haired, blue-eyed Irish-pale girl—but

I soon see she is trying to make a point. *Terrible, non?* She says, taking the offending scarf away.

Now you choose.

I feel like this is a trick question. I like red. Actually, I love red. I have loved it since I was a little girl and wore a red cotton shift dress to school practically every day—or at least as many times during the week that I could get away with. I wore this red dress by itself during the summertime as a sleeveless shift, and then during the winter it served as a jumper. I wore it over a white blouse, and another white blouse that had little red polka dots, and during the winter, over a black turtleneck. Even to this day, red and black is my favorite combination. I read that in feng shui it's the color combination of luck and power. Anyway, I've been wearing red for as long as I can remember. Plus, I wear red lipstick. Bright red lipstick. It can go in or out of style, and I don't care. I will wear red lipstick. I started wearing it because of my friend Brigitte, whom I met in London right after college. She wore red lipstick. She was an incredibly artsy and beautiful girl. She gave me a tube of red lipstick she bought at Marks & Spencer, and I have never looked back. Well, that's not exactly true, because once in a while, I will have a crisis in confidence and ask my husband if he thinks I should switch to something less showy, but he always says no, I should wear my red lipstick because it makes me happy.

Still, standing in this shop with a real French woman watching me as I hold up a bright red scarf, I wonder what she will say. She stands back and considers me and my relationship to the color red.

I look in the mirror and I see myself—a woman who is perhaps trying just a little too hard. What is this thing with red? Why do I cling to it? It's not the red lipstick or Brigitte or even the little red dress from my childhood; it's something else. But the thought of giving it up worries me and yet, I see what's about to happen. Micheline purses her lips, shakes her head, and quietly says, *Non.*

No? No to red, no to the red lipstick? No to this dream of what red means to me? But before I can ask these things, she picks up a blue scarf, places it under my chin, and turns me to face the mirror and smiles. Ah, yes. I must admit, I let out a deep sigh, because the truth is right there in front of me. Blue is my color. I look good in blue. I look peaceful and calm and, dare I say, confident. Oh, and I should say, this is not some timid pastel ice blue. This is a deep Atlantic Ocean blue. This is the blue of my French grandmother's family, who sailed over in the sixteenth century from their homeland in Normandy and made their way to the new land of Canada. This is a dangerous blue. A brave blue. A royal blue. A rugged blue. An adventurous blue. Perhaps, I think, blue is the new red!

Micheline seems very pleased with herself.

We frolic through the store, looking for more blue. Blue dresses, blue sweaters, blue skirts, blue trousers. It is a lot of fun. The ladies who run the shop seem to know Micheline, and so they don't mind the fact that we are taking so very long to select something. Here's what I love about shops in France, and actually in most of Europe. The salesladies are truly knowledgeable about the clothing. They are not working in a shop, just biding time until a Hollywood director discovers them. No, this is a very respectable career and they take their jobs quite seriously. You can trust them to steer you toward the kinds of colors, fabrics, and styles that suit you. Oh, and often everything is organized by color. And everything is *very* organized. They are not bunched together but very elegantly displayed. Still, as I get more serious about actually buying something, I notice the little price tags. Things are expensive. Micheline picks out a short-sleeved cobalt blue sweater dress for me. Actually it's not exactly a dress, but something you would wear over a black, fitted top. Or a turtleneck. That's what I imagine. It costs almost 200 euros. I am not going to buy this dress. I know this immediately. First of all, there's the price, and second of all, I'm worried about it fitting into my suitcase and then my having to lug it all over France.

I say no to the dress. I am being practical.

However, when it comes to a bright blue feather boa—yes, something a dancer in the Folies Bergères would wear—well, that's a different story. I prance around the store with the feather boa. I take a photo of myself in front of the mirror with the feather boa. Everyone agrees it's quite spectacular. Micheline smiles, but I can see she is being indulgent. She would prefer I buy the sweater dress. Something sensible. After all, she is used to working with businesspeople. But, I'm not a businessperson, so why should I be sensible?!

I buy the feather boa. Because that's just the kind of gal I am. And besides, it's blue. So that's some progress.

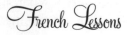

Find your signature color. And if you've already got a signature color, consider that it may be time to change it. Yes, it's important to decide what colors look best on you, but more than this, consider which colors make you feel more like yourself. It's never too late to take risks, to reinvent yourself. Ask yourself, what do you want from life?

What is your true aim and purpose? This actually has more to do with fashion, beauty, and style than you might imagine. French women believe that beauty comes from the inside, rather than from the outside, so why not look into your heart to get in touch with your true beauty? Begin to see yourself as the heroine of your own life.

This true identity might not emerge immediately for you, but if you take time each day to enjoy your own beauty, little by little you will reconnect with your essential self and your unique look will light up.

If you can afford it and have the space, invest in a full-length three-way mirror. It's a remarkable thing and allows you to see yourself as others see you. It'll also give you the feeling of looking at yourself objectively, as if you are an actress in a movie—and the star of your own life—because you are!

Be willing to "changer les idées". This is a French expression for changing your ideas, but it goes deeper than that. It means to clear your mind and reconsider a new possibility. French women do this on a daily basis by switching up the route they take to work, or buying groceries at a new market, but they also "changer les idées" as a way to refresh and spice up ordinary life. And they do this on a daily basis, rather than waiting until a big day when they go through one huge transformation involving major surgery and buckets of money.

Rather, be willing to change a little every day. Take risks. And finally, consider adding some much-needed blue (or green or pink or brown or yellow or violet) to your wardrobe.

CHAPTER THREE

⁓

I Took My Troubles Down to Madame Rue

There is a certain age when a woman must be beautiful
to be loved and then there comes a time when she
must be loved to be beautiful.

—FRANÇOISE SAGAN

TODAY I AM meeting an American expat friend at the famous café, Les Deux Magots on the Left Bank. It's a big, touristy place, but very central to any Left Bank excursion into the world of French beauty, skincare, and the art of *être bien dans sa peau*. Feeling good in one's own skin and being comfortable with oneself.

My friend's name is Heather Stimmler-Hall.

In a way, her name says it all. There is something about that hyphenated last name that makes one think of upper-crust American girls whose great-great-great-grandmothers came over on the Mayflower. Girls who attended Miss Porter's

School and went on to study at Bryn Mawr. Oh, and then there is the first name—Heather. Much more modern. Young. It doesn't exactly go with the hyphenated last name, but then again, it doesn't *not* go. It adds a little dash of something wild. Unpredictable. As if on the day of her birth, her parents had a Greenwich Village moment and spontaneously took it upon themselves to go against the family tradition, bypass the obvious waspy names her cousins were given— forgo the Polly, Page, and Piper—and name their newborn baby girl Heather.

All this is a flight of imagination on my part. Heather is actually from Arizona, but she still looks and holds herself like a New England beauty with great cheekbones, a fierce intelligence, and beauty to boot! Here's the delightful thing about Heather. She's aware of the impression she makes on people and so she approaches every encounter with grace and elegance, yes. But also, a healthy dose of humor.

In fact, there's even a bit of naughtiness in the middle of all this elegance. Still, it's so subtle, you have to really be on your toes to catch it.

I met Heather a few years ago when her book *Naughty Paris: A Lady's Guide to the Sexy City* first came out. I was actually introduced to her by Ethan Gilsdorf, author of the book *Fantasy Freaks and Gaming Geeks.* We were on a panel together at the Muse and the Marketplace conference in Boston not too long ago. Yes, I know, French women authors and dwellers of the imaginary realm—strange bedfellows!

Still, he told me I must meet his friend, Heather. And so I did. First in New York City and later in Paris. Heather leads tours for groups, individuals, women-only, and everything in between. She owns and operates a tour service called Secrets of Paris. Oh, and did I mention she's tall and slender and very stylish? Well, she is.

I am coming from the 17th arrondisement, where I have been visiting my friend Nancy, and so while the clouds were merely threatening a rainfall when I walked into the Métro, by the time I come out at Mabillon near Saint Germain-des-Prés, the sky has turned pitch-black and the rain is pouring down. I've never seen anything quite like it. So volatile and so sudden. I can't help thinking this is a very French rain. Passionate, insistent, and yet mysterious. On the Boulevard St. Germaine there is an explosion of colorful umbrellas. Surprisingly, they are much more colorful than anything you'd see in New York. I hardly see any generic black umbrellas, and I remember how my French tutor, Marceline, said you should only buy a bright umbrella so that your spirits will be lifted on a dark, rainy day.

Unfortunately, I have not brought any umbrella—colorful or otherwise. And so, I crowd into the little space at the stairs at the entrance to the Métro, hoping for a break in the rain. I am shoulder to shoulder with all these Parisians and tourists, and we are jostled even closer together every time someone comes into the Métro. Still, the French are very good-natured about the whole thing and seem to actually enjoy this sudden turn of events.

I, of course, am anxious. I don't want to be late for my meeting, but somehow being around all these very happy people, I find myself relaxing. The sky is streaked with lightning and suddenly there is a huge clap of thunder, and you know what the lady and man next to me do? They laugh! *C'est la vie!* Yes, they are actually thrilled by the forces of nature, the power the weather has to change our so-called important human plans. And so I relax and wait. And before you know it, the storm has passed and I cross the boulevard to find Heather waiting for me in front of the café under an awning.

She is wearing a proper, but very chic, ensemble. A tweedy skirt, a black cashmere sweater, and a classic trench, along with a little rain hat. Oh, and she remembered to bring her umbrella. Sensible girl, I think, but then I notice the lace-up boots and I realize that she hasn't forgot her naughty side, either.

We walk around the little outdoor tables, and then once inside, we order two *chocolat chauds*. Yes, it's hot chocolate, but so much richer than our hot chocolate at home. Think less milk, more chocolate. And all served in a silver pitcher with a lovely china cup and saucer. Heather tells me our first stop will be to interview her esthetician, Véronique. And so before too long, we leave the café, and since the rain has started up once again, I share her umbrella. We dash across the boulevard and down a few side streets, until we get to 3 rue de Buci in the 6th arrondisement. Along the way, since this is the Latin Quarter and very old, we negotiate over a couple of cobblestone paths, doing our best to avoid the puddles.

And then, here we are—we have arrived at Institut Esthétique Buci. We ring a discreet doorbell, and then we climb a couple of steps, walk across a courtyard where I can see into other office buildings through glassed-in windows, and finally come upon the office—or I should say the salon. Although, it is nothing like any salon I've been to in the States. It feels more as if I've entered someone's private home. My friend Nancy, who has lived in Paris since the 1980s and is married to a French man, says that traditionally shops, offices, and *ateliers* (workshops) are inside an individual's home. In fact, her husband is a doctor and his office is in their home.

Nancy tells me that this creates a much more intimate environment. And because of this, French women are used to getting a lot of personal attention. This carries over to all aspects of their lives, from doctor visits to leg waxing to selecting a dress or new shoes or planning a dinner party and even going to the market to buy some cheese. For the French, it's all about the interaction, the relationship between people. That's why it's considered very rude to walk into a French shop and not say *Bonjour!* And engage in a little chitchat. To walk in wordlessly and start fingering the goods would be equivalent to walking into your neighbor's house without saying anything and start making yourself a cup of tea in her kitchen. I think this is where we get confused by the French. As Americans, we're all about independence and self-service, but the French are all about inter-relatedness and service. Service is everything!

And so, when I meet Véronique, I am not surprised by how much time she spends with Heather and me talking about her work. This woman, in her lovely pink lab coat, brings us into her office and asks if we'd like a glass of Perrier. She is not one of those incredibly skinny French women, but rather she is a little curvy. Just a little. And she has short, stylish blond hair.

Véronique has owned Institut Esthétique Buci for over twenty years. In this time, she has watched as her first clients have grown up, married, and had children. And now, these clients' daughters also come to see her. *I am closer to my clients than a hairdresser,* she explains to me. *Because, for example, waxing is so private.*

Heather adds that French women don't shave. It's too stubbly, not soft. Waxing is the thing here. When I ask Véronique about the different intimate waxing services she provides, she tells me that the Brazilian wax is always popular, but there's also *Jardin a la Français,* which is also called the French Wax. It means a little triangle is left and not much more. In France, they use this pink bubblegum-looking wax to remove unwanted hair. It looks quite different from our green wax, and I am told that it hurts less. I ask Véronique about other spa services, such as manicures and pedicures, but she tells me that while French women do go in for these services, they are more likely to get regular facials and massages. Most French women either do their nails at home or don't use polish at all.

Next I learn about the lymphatic drainage massage. It's very popular in France. In fact, it was created by a French man back in the early 1930s in the French Riviera and is said to help the circulation of lymph through the body. As I talk to more and more French women, I hear this recurring theme relating to the idea of releasing something. Some French women tell me they have seen therapists who specialize in releasing past life traumas, and some have told me they have had their "aura cleansed." And now, I am learning about lymph circulation. While I'm not sure what it all means, I do know on an instinctual level that this release or flow must be part of the secret to the French woman's ability to maintain her sense of balance. Perhaps it doesn't give her *ooh la la* per se, but I wonder if it allows her to open the door to *ooh la la.*

When I ask about cosmetic surgery, Véronique shakes her head in disapproval. Heather whispers something like *French women don't do plastic.* Rather, a French woman will age naturally, but do whatever she can to feel beautiful. Not young, but beautiful, Véronique explains. *It's better, no? More natural?*

Véronique tells me that she has always been interested in beauty and skincare. When she was a little girl, she actually took all her dolls and removed their makeup and wiped their faces free of all color. Then she experimented with different looks, using her mother's makeup. Her advice on makeup is quite simple—"whatever you do, don't over-do it." She tells me that French women don't tend to use injectables or facial fillers. The truth is, we all have a plethora of skincare potions and possibilities, however for the French woman it's all about pleasure and what *feels* good. So facials, massages, creams, and lotions are the way to go. And like many estheticians, Véronique sells her own line of skincare products in her salon.

I ask if she sees any major differences between a French woman's makeup and an American's and she tells me that *American women want to look good from a distance. French women also want to look good up close, and more importantly, they want to be touchable.* This seems like an obvious statement, but when I consider some of our American celebrities' penchant for cosmetic surgery, I can't help thinking that they look great from a distance, or in a magazine photograph that's been photoshopped, but whenever I see a woman who's had work done, there is something rather frozen and untouchable about her. And then there's the very expression, "work done." The French will always choose something pleasurable over "work." This is why seasonable visits to the spas are so important.

Véronique pauses for a moment, crosses her legs, and then leans forward and lowers her voice. *French women want to look good for our husbands. We want to keep them,* she whispers.

Heather nods in agreement.

I wonder about this. Is it a concern for American women, too? Somehow I don't think American women worry about keeping their man quite so much once they're married. But then again, maybe we should. Maybe French women know something about human nature—or I should say the nature of men—that we don't know, or would rather not know?

I notice Véronique sneak a peek at my wedding band and then she continues, her eyes meeting mine. *Never do less once you are married. Maybe do more.*

I shake my head in agreement, solemnly taking in her words of wisdom.

After all, my husband is in Australia, on the other side of the world, measuring coral and researching sea level rise. We are both at work in our different ways, but as I listen to Véronique talk about love and sensuality and how taking care of one's body and feeling good in one's skin are integral to keeping love alive—I feel a kind of aching in my body.

There is not a whole lot of time to dwell on this, because Heather and I are off to our next appointment. We are going to Herboristerie D'Hippocrate on 42, rue Saint André des Arts, and so we have a short walk. The rain has stopped now and we make our way down the winding alleyways. I am wearing my little pointy ballet flats and they tend to get slippery on the wet cobblestones, so I find myself walking very carefully, struggling to keep up with the long-legged, highly energetic Heather.

You will love this place, she tells me as she opens a heavy wooden door that tinkles from the sound of a little bell at the entryway. The place has a slightly Harry Potter feel to it. The room is dark, filled with dark wood and shelves with hundreds—maybe thousands—of little brown bottles. It takes a few seconds before my eyes adjust to the light or lack of light. There is a velvet curtain at the back of the store, and it is being slowly opened. An older woman comes forward, greeting us with a solemn *Bonjour!*

Heather and I exchange pleasantries with her and then Heather tells her about her stomach difficulties. She needs to cleanse things. I'm not sure exactly what this means. She is speaking quickly in French, and I am losing ground. I actually don't mind this because it gives me an opportunity to let my mind drift into a kind of dream, a fantasy. This place, with its bottles with pretty names in French, seems to be a kind of good witch's house. The little bottles all have white labels on them, and the names and purposes of the herbs and liquids are written in black ink. And then I see a bottle labeled TONIQUE SEXUEL.

Maybe it's just me—but whenever I see the word "sexual" my interest is immediately aroused. And if you spell it the French way, well, doubly so. Heather and the herbalist approach me and ask if I want to buy something. Well, of course I do. I want some of this Tonique Sexuel—for the bottle, for the label, for the idea of it, for the notion that I will return home with a little brown bottle of Love Potion No. 9, *a la française!*

Mais, oui (but, yes) the madame says, *Bien sur!* And before I know it, she is in the back room and Heather and I are spying on her through the velvet curtain as she mixes a fresh batch of Tonique Sexuel for me, using several different bottles and combining the ingredients. She brings it out with her and allows me to see it before she seals the jar closed with the cap. It looks a little like apple juice. In fact, it smells like apple juice that was a bit fermented. Something you might get drunk on. Wow. My imagination takes a little leap into the air, does a sexy pirouette, and lands on pink ballet-slippered tippy toes at the cash register. That'll be thirty euros or about forty-five dollars, and I pay for it feeling so happy, as if I am Harry Potter himself and I've just entered the Chamber of Secrets. Imagine, for a mere forty-five dollars you will feel very hot and sexy and your libido will never be quite the same. *Ooh la la!*

And yet, to be honest with you, I know I will never actually take even a tiny teaspoon of this Tonique Sexuel because, truth be told, I am afraid I might end up like the man in that song "Love Potion No. 9" and I'd start running around Paris kissing every man in sight! But, I like the bottle. I like the label and the experience. I'm kind of an experience junkie, which has occasionally got me into some tight spots.

From here, Heather takes me to Métro Concord to the Right Bank, where we walk down the rue de Rivoli and shop. Heather and I go into a shoe store and she tries on a pair of thigh-high platform lace-up boots. They're from Italy, made of beautiful leather, and cost a fortune. Heather cannot afford them. I certainly cannot afford them, but there's this part of me that thinks I should buy them for her. I should take a quick swig of the Tonique Sexuel and buy the boots and while I'm at it, buy a pair for myself and go strutting down along the Siene, waving to all the tourist boats going by, singing *"La Vie en Rose."* That's how powerful I feel!

French Lessons

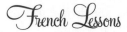

French women have an expression, "prendre soin de soi," which means to take good care of oneself. This means treating your body well, getting regular massages and other treatments that make you feel beautiful. French women believe in maintenance and taking care of their God-given gifts. So, you will never find a French woman who's "let herself go." You won't find French TV shows that feature huge, eye-popping physical transformations, because French women do little things, every day.

Take a look at your beauty regime and see if there's a balance between things that make you just look good and things that make you feel good. While a great massage and salt scrub might not be as flashy and obvious as a new nail color, it goes a long way in terms of feeling connected to your own body. And when you feel connected to your own body, you feel more sensual.

French women are very individualistic when it comes to their beauty routines—some will spritz Evian water on their face every day and others are loyal to certain face creams or scrubs—however, all French women develop the lifelong habit of taking care of themselves. This isn't about "looking" good (although that will be an end result). It's about feeling good. Feeling touchable. And when you feel touchable, your love life gets a big boost as well. So, you won't need to go to an herbalist and buy yourself a bottle of Tonique Sexuel, because you will feel sexy from the inside out.

!!!

CHAPTER FOUR

The Sensuous Woman

One is not born, but rather becomes, a woman.
—SIMONE DE BEAUVOIR

TODAY I MEET with Patricia Gellenter. The sun has come out again and I am standing just outside the rue Monges Métro. I have scheduled a special Indian massage with Patricia Gellenter. She's the daughter of my friend Terrence Gellenter, an expat who's been living in Paris for many years. He recommended that I talk to Patricia about French women and beauty and skincare, because she is a wealth of information; so here I am.

Patricia is not actually French. She's from Spain, but she has lived in Paris for quite a long time, so she's full of opinions about French women and happy to share them with me.

Setting up this meeting has been an adventure. Maybe even a drama. First, we e-mailed back and forth several times. Once we established the time and the date, it took several more e-mails to get to where we would meet. But finally, it is agreed. Métro Monge. Ten thirty. I come up from the Métro, right on time, and Patricia is nowhere to be seen. I wait. I people watch. And about fifteen minutes later, she arrives. She is a very pretty young woman. Possibly in her early thirties, but she could also be in her late twenties. She has long dark hair that she's pulled back into a casual chignon. This is the look for lots of women in France. It's one of those hairstyles that looks elegant and chic, and yet unplanned, and you get this sense that she would only need to pull out just one strategic hair pin and then all those luscious curls would come tumbling down around her shoulders. *Tres romantique!* (very romantic!)

As we walk down the street, she tells me something that I find interesting and even a little bit funny. *Look at this.* She points out she is carrying her handbag just so. *I always carry my bag like it's a little basket on the crook of my arm. This way is more ladylike,* she tells me. *Also, everyone can see how pretty your bag is.*

Unfortunately, I am not carrying the kind of handbag you can carry on the crook of your arm. My bag goes over the shoulder and across my chest and is tightly zippered in case I run into some purse-stealing thugs on the Métro. Still, I must admit there is something to this other way of carrying a bag. It looks so much more ladylike and sexy and actually does remind me of a woman carrying a basket to the market.

I wonder about the idea of how being ladylike and how being watchful and even a little bit wary does not always go hand in hand, and I remember how my friend's husband, Jean Pierre, carries Beatrice's bag over his shoulder when they walk through the sketchy parts of town in Toulouse. It's interesting that our American men don't seem to be okay with carrying our bags.

However, I don't have too much time to contemplate this because we have arrived at the French "gym." I have to laugh at this. I am so used to American gyms, where you walk into a huge warehouse-like space with what seems like hundreds of machines lined up in front of television sets, accompanied by the sound of grinding treadmills and the whoosh of elliptical machines, the boom-boom-boom of cross-trainers pounding against rubber. The whirling of spinning stationary bikes. The feeling that you have entered an alternate universe where strength and power and sweat is everything and the one who sweats the most and breathes the heaviest wins.

This French gym is empty. Well, not completely empty, but there is only one man—a very handsome, very slender French man—dressed all in black, standing behind a black lacquer reception desk, looking slightly peeved, and there are several machines in this gym.

True, in the center of the room, there are about ten or eleven pristine-looking stationary bikes, but that's it. Interestingly enough, they are all facing one another, spaced evenly into a perfect little circle. Also, the lighting is really lovely. Kind of moody. And the windows are made to be reflective, so it feels as if you're looking out at a series of smoky mirrors. And there is soft jazz playing in the background. Honestly, I feel as if we've entered a fancy restaurant and people are about to order an aperitif, rather than getting geared up for a sweat-inducing cardiovascular workout.

Only, as I said, there are no people. Patricia explains to me that the gym just opened up and that this concept of going to a place with machines is new to the French. *Dance is one thing,* she tells me, *because it's artistic and intellectual, but generally the French don't like to get sweaty in groups.*

This is so interesting to me, because I think part of the reason people go to gyms is to exercise within the context of a group of people who are doing the same thing. Although, this is exactly why I don't like going to the gym. You get on the StairMaster or the treadmill and you huff and puff and sweat, and there's these burly guys huffing and puffing right next to you. It feels just a tad too intimate to me and too close. And I think I'm a lot like French women; I'm not crazy about sweating. And when I do sweat, I like to do it in private. Or, only with one other person. In the bedroom. With my husband.

I do love dance classes and I admit they make me sweat, but they also make me smile and laugh. French women don't trust any kind of exercise that involves a lot of sweat and makes your face grimace. French women don't believe in that. They do have *"Les sports,"* but this will involve something delightful and artful, without too much suffering.

Despite this, Patricia tells me that gyms are beginning to pop up in France—mostly in Paris for now, but they're completely different from the gym rat phenomenon we have in America. I do believe our gyms are masculine. That's the ethos. They are utilitarian, rough, and noisy places—men and women mingle—and it's not easy to escape the sounds of burly men grunting. True, sometimes American gyms will confine the men who lift heavy weights to something they call the "cage." But you can see them and hear them. When they are leaving the gym, with their enormous biceps bursting out of their T-shirts that announce their affiliation to some team, they will eye you there on the gravitron. There you are, hanging, praying that you can fight off the upper arm weakness, and they will look at you and flex a muscle as if to say, *Yeah, I'm bigger and stronger than you are, babe! I'm a man.*

And sometimes I wonder, are we in some kind of crazy

competition with them? Is it possible that the more toned we get, the buffer we get, the more successful we are, the more men need to pump themselves up? And how far will we go with this competition? This face-off in the middle of Bally's?

The French don't worry about this. Although, I will admit I sometimes wonder if they're in an opposite kind of competition with women, which is who can be the skinniest. And as far as I can see—at least among the younger generation—the boys are winning. Still, they're not competing inside the gym. French men and French women just don't work out together. And French men do not get pumped up. The man at the reception desk is evidence of that. Nobody seems to worry about getting pumped up. And there's very little competition between men and women.

I follow Patricia down the stairs to the dressing rooms. Again, I must adjust my eyes to the mood lighting. She leads me to a room where there is a massage table and soft music playing. She lights a few fragrant candles and then asks me to undress and lie on the table between the sheets. It's interesting to me that there is no separate dressing room, no little locker for my purse, no robe. It's very straightforward. Take off your clothes and get under the sheets. I have heard from my French friends that office visits to the doctor are like this. You undress right there in front of the doctor. It's assumed that you're not embarrassed or shy or afraid of some untoward collision between the professional and the personal.

Still, I feel very relaxed with Patricia. Somehow, her voice and demeanor make me feel secure. As I lie on the table, she asks me if I have any medical issues, anything I'd like to tell her. And I tell her that I'm fine, except I feel a cold coming on and I'm just exhausted. I've been racing around so much. She listens intently, nods her head, and smiles with great sympathy. She suggests I take *"curuma"* for my bones. This is tumeric. I make a mental note. I close my eyes. I know my massage will be lovely, but it will probably not be enough for me. What I really need is a week at a spa. I am that tired.

Patricia begins with my scalp and gives me a deep massage. Unfortunately, I just had a "brush out" (the French expression for a shampoo and blow-dry) the day before, but *c'est la vie.*

And the massage oil has a delicious aroma. I ask Patricia what it is and she whispers it has almond and jasmine oils. She spends a long time on my scalp—apparently, this can be the source of all sorts of medical issues. From here she works on my spine, shoulders, arms, legs, back, and then surprisingly—my stomach. Yes, she rubs and presses and manipulates my belly. I must admit I'm a little nervous about this. I've never received a massage that includes the abdomen, but what the heck, I'm in France!

Afterward, I feel heavenly. I smell great, but I'm still sticky when I put on my clothes. There's no shower available and Patricia says it would be a shame to remove all those wonderful oils from my skin. Oh, and one look in the mirror—I see my straight blown-out hair is completely wild! I look like some kind of lioness with reddish-blond curls standing straight out. I do my best to tame it, but Patricia says she likes it and I should always wear my hair like that. *That's your essence,* she tells me. And I am not sure if she is being honest or making fun of me. But then, I think maybe it is my essence and maybe I am a little wild and curly haired. Maybe I should stop blow-drying it straight and let it go natural. Perhaps all the energy I devote to tamping down this wildness is what has exhausted me.

And then, we are off again. This time to the Ile Saint-Louis where we find a café overlooking the Seine. We order some tea. Actually, she drinks tea—herbal—and I have a *café au lait*, because I have yet to give up dairy like the rest of the planet. I ask Patricia about the gym and why it was so empty. She tells me that the French prefer to do gymnastics *because it's graceful and feminine*. She continues, *French women know how to take care of themselves. They don't worry so much about being perfect. American women overdo it. They focus too much on sports. They run too much*. When I ask her for beauty advice, she tells me that it's important to stop worrying about being perfect. *Take care of yourself. Find a good color. Don't eat so much. Develop your personality. Dress for yourself.* As far as beauty tips go, Patricia's advice is very down-to-earth. She tells me that she wakes up each morning and drinks hot water with lemon. She'll make facial masques using egg white, honey, and yogurt. She massages her face with rosewater and puts ice water under her eyes if they get puffy.

I ask her how she stays so slim and she tells me that she eats smaller portions, fresh foods, and doesn't snack. For exercise? She walks. Any suggestions on losing weight? Patricia tells me that regular massages are key. No surprise here, since she is a masseuse, but then she adds that French women will either go to the *Hammam*, a North African–style bath that's not very expensive, and you can stay the whole day there, or they'll "take the waters" in spas in the country. Normandy and Evian are popular destinations, but there are little spas all along the coastline of France. The idea is that seawater has healing powers and so men and women will go for a day or several days and get seaweed wraps, mud baths, and enjoy the waters. It's called Thalassotherapy. All the French women go after they have a baby, according to my friend Nancy. And many go three or four times a year. It's all about relaxation, and there's virtually no exercising at these spas, but rather they go to detox and de-stress. They lounge around all day in their robes and swim and get massages and well, just relax! This sounds exactly like something I need.

I make a promise to myself to go and get some of those healing powers for myself. It's been years since I got a mud bath or a seaweed wrap or soaked in a hot spring filled with magnesium and calcium. As Patricia continues, my mind drifts to a memory of me in New Mexico, soaking in the pool at Ojo Caliente. It was before the place was bought and turned into a resort and spa. It was just a ragtag group of small adobe structures surrounded by a series of natural hot springs. Very down-to-earth, but very sensual. I was staying in an artist colony in Taos the summer of 2002 and my husband, then my boyfriend, was in New York City. We didn't do Internet in those days, not really, and so every day I would go to the mailbox to find a handwritten letter from him. They were pretty steamy, as I recall. And just as I am falling into these memories, I am pulled back into the present moment, when Patricia tells me *and of course making love is very good.*

Good for what? I ask.

Beauty. Health. That's the French woman's secret. That's how she stays so slim!

Ah, so this is the secret! I solemnly nod my head and make a vow to pay more attention to my husband when I get home.

French Lessons

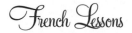

Get yourself a massage. Even if you just do it for your birthday, you'll feel the difference. French women will often get a massage in preparation for each new season. And if you can't afford it, take a class on partner massage, so you can give and receive.

Consider letting your own natural essence loose. Perhaps it's your wild hair or your quirky smile or perhaps your loud laugh. Be completely yourself.

And finally, if you don't like the gym, don't go. Find something that makes you feel beautiful and happy and gives you a great workout. Try Zumba (a personal favorite). Oh, and did you know they now have Zumba Gold for women of a certain age? Well, they do! There's also Zumba Toning where you use strength-building weights. J'adore! Consider walking more. Eating less. Take up yoga. And enjoy the feeling of inhabiting your own body.

Finally, carry your bag on the crook of your arm, as if you were a lady just coming home from the market with a pile of the season's freshest, most delectable peaches. And if it's too heavy, see if you can get your man to help you out!

!!!

CHAPTER FIVE

The Pleasure Principle

The most beautiful makeup for a woman is passion.
—YVES SAINT LAURENT

FOR AN AUTHOR of a new book, it's one of those moments you dream about.

You walk into a party where there's another author—more famous than you—surrounded by acolytes, which makes sense; she is, after all, teaching a weeklong writing workshop and this is the final celebratory party. This famous writer—she is ignoring you. Not being particularly friendly, not that there's some big reason for her to be all that interested in you. After all, you are just the guest of one of her acolytes. But, still.

You walk out onto the terrace. It's a balmy night in Paris and your friend—the acolyte—introduces you to a former student of the famous writer. And this woman, sitting there serenely with her four-month-old baby nestled against her chest, looks at you and exclaims—*oh, I love your book! It's wonderful! I can't believe I'm sitting next to you!*

This sort of thing rarely happens to me. And so, I am all ears as this young woman begins singing my praises. Okay, not singing my praises—singing my book's praises—which actually, at this point, feels like something somebody else wrote, say a distant cousin, about ten years ago, while she was living in another country.

And this gal—this pretty late twenty/early thirty-something American named Sylvia who has been living in France for the last several years—wants to help me! She introduces me to her husband who is sitting beside her, now holding their baby, and then she tells me how much she adores Paris and the fresh produce markets, the parks, the architecture, the lingerie! She is so pretty—this willowy girl with her long dark hair. She asks me where I am staying while in Paris and I tell her that I am currently with a friend in Vanves, but will soon be back to Paris in a few days. Sylvia asks me if I have a place to stay when I get back. Actually, no. And so she invites me to stay in her home in the very tony 17th arrondisement.

And tony it is! A week later, I am lugging my bags up to the wrought iron gate on a hilly street overlooking the Eiffel Tower. The building is one of those late-eighteenth-century Haussman deals with an imposing front and a gorgeous, red-carpeted lobby. I ring for the concierge, who is located in a little apartment just outside the front door. She directs me to the elevator—a tiny cage decorated with gold leaf curlicues. I maneuver myself and my luggage into the little cage. Honestly, I do believe you simply cannot get fat in France, because if you do, you will not fit into their elevators, you will not be able to sit in the little Métro seats or fit into the little airplane-size bathrooms, and you certainly won't be able to negotiate all those narrow, winding stairs. And so, I stand tall as I ascend to the fourth floor, which is really the fifth floor, but that's another story.

Sylvia greets me at the door, holding her baby in her arms in a kind of white linen sling contraption. She has the dreamy look and disposition of a woman who is still in the throes of new motherhood. I believe it's a calm they get from sitting for long stretches of time, their baby at their breast, listening to the little gurgling sounds and staring out the window. Sylvia, barefoot, instructs me to take off my shoes, which I do, and then she leads me to her living room.

Windows.

Lots of them.

Curved.

Floor to ceiling.

With a close-up, panoramic view of the Eiffel Tower, posing in front of gorgeous white clouds. It's like I'm in a 3-D postcard overlooking a brilliant blue day in Paris. Well, it is in 3-D because here I am and there it is, seemingly inches away. Really, I feel as if I could just reach out the window and grab hold of a column of the steel from that *Tour Eiffel* and pull it into my chest, holding it close, quickly catching my breath before I give it a great big friendly American hug. *Thanks for the Statue of Liberty,* I would say if I could actually talk to it.

Good thing Sylvia is such a dreamy girl, because she seems completely unfazed by my reverie. Ah, new motherhood. I do remember those days, but it's been a long, long time and in fact, not too long ago, my daughter married a wonderful fellow. Soon the cycle will begin again and I will be a grandmother. But for now, I am simply a *femme d'un certain âge,* traipsing around France while my second husband digs for corals on the beaches of Western Australia. With all this life experience, you'd think I would get over being constantly, breathlessly enthralled by France. But somehow I'm not. Somehow, I cannot get enough. I envy Sylvia, an American mother, living here and experiencing firsthand what it is like to have a baby in a country that is famous for its talent of raising children who don't throw their food. Not that my daughter ever threw her food.

Well, actually, she probably did throw her food, but I have long forgotten about that. She is twenty-seven, after all.

In any event, I am here to stay with Sylvia and learn about her life in Paris. I'm especially interested in how she's been able to keep her *ooh la la* after having a baby. Oh, and she also has a three-year-old boy, so you know she's a very busy woman. Here's the impressive thing about Sylvia—despite the fact that she just had her second child, she's in amazing shape. She meditates and practices yoga. She's writing a memoir, and more than this, she has just signed up for a course in what the French call physiotherapy—or vaginal rejuvenation—which is something most new mothers in France receive after giving birth and is paid for by the French government.

We are standing in her kitchen and she is making us a cup of tea when she tells me she's very interested in finding out what the fuss is all about. *Because,* she begins, *I really want to explore the authentic French life and this is part of it. It's important.*

So, you're going to make an appointment? I ask, taking the cup of tea from her and sitting down by the counter.

Oh yes, she tells me, and she offers me a cookie, but then she has to leave the room because her toddler has woken up from his afternoon nap.

When she returns, she tells me that she'll e-mail me a description of the experience if I want to write about it, since it definitely relates to *ooh la la.*

And I say, oh, yes, please let me know. And then we are onto other things. Sylvia tells me about her book and about her experiences traveling the world, before she was married and moved to France. I have a wonderful stay with her and spend a good deal of my time staring out her window.

And then, several weeks later, I receive an e-mail from Sylvia, describing post-childbirth treatments. By this time, I have been all over France learning about the secret of *ooh la la* from all different sorts of women, but still, this e-mail is really fascinating. So fascinating, in fact, that I ask Sylvia if I can include it here and she says, yes, absolutely. So here is what she says:

So—this is what it's like. I walk into this office and the waiting room is filled with women. Of all ages. Young and old. New mothers and grandmothers, too. It's always packed. The walls are covered with beautiful art of women's bodies. It looks like an old doctor's office from the sixties that some Freudian-loving therapist decorated. Each session lasts around twenty minutes, and generally you go in for ten sessions.

The first time I went, I was fairly surprised at how— well, intimate it is. A lovely therapist, a woman, has you lie down on a table, and she simply gets her fingers into you and asks you to start squeezing your pelvic muscles. Kegels. But not just simple Kegels—really fancy ones. Kegels where you tighten up as much as you can, release a little, then tighten again. Kegels where you stand up and lift a leg, walk in place. Kegels where you lie down and do sit-ups. And this entire time, this blessed woman's fingers are inside of you, pressing onto little points and working with the muscles. It's pretty incredible.

During ten minutes of the session, you take out your "electric dildo," which is your own personal piece of equipment that you pick up in a pharmacy with a prescription from a doctor! The dildo gets plugged in and placed inside you. You start doing your Kegels as this, well, electrical thing begins to pulse. A computer screen gives you biofeedback and lets you know how you are doing.

They say, technically, that this therapy is supposed to help you not "leak urine." Which can happen after pregnancy or with age. But honestly, I wasn't leaking and I don't think most women are leaking who are in there. They are doing this therapy to get that area tightened up, to get those juices flowing, to get the zap back. I think that everyone says it is for "urine" so that the government will keep paying for it. Or the insurance companies will pay for it. It's a bit of a French fib.

When I asked my therapist why this doesn't exist in the United States, she simply told me, "Too puritanical a society."

As for me, I certainly am not too puritanical. In fact, I am just about to throw away my post pregnancy granny panties and switch back into my fancy ones.

I simply have to ask—why, oh why, oh why do new mothers in America not get this!? Rather, I know from personal experience that we are sent home from the hospital after a day or two, newborn in tow, and when we get our first ob/gyn examination, the doctor says, nonchalantly, *doing your Kegels?* I don't know about you, but nobody ever gave me much instruction or encouragement regarding *my Kegels.*

Post birth, all the emphasis seems to be on the baby. And I loved my baby just as much as the next full-blooded American gal, but from the distance of a fifty-something-year-old with a larger view of the world, I would say, perhaps—no, not perhaps—we should definitely take a little more time on making sure mama's body gets back to its pre-pregnancy shape.

In America, we do care about the outside shape of mama's body. We have big glossy photographs of our movie stars on the cover of all our women's and entertainment magazines, touting how Jessica or Reese or Julia or Kate got that post-pregnancy bod back into a bikini and wow, aren't they looking hot?! And so, while there is all this emphasis on the external, we seem to forget about the parts of a woman that are not seen, that are invisible to the world—that is, until we hit our fifties and Whoopi Goldberg tells us that we should buy some Depends for our "spritzing" problems.

I should explain that in America we have something called *surgical laser* vaginal rejuvenation, but I just can't help thinking this is another example of waiting until things are really at the point of no return and then fixing the problem in one big and expensive procedure that actually does nothing to educate the individual woman and connect her to the power she possesses to care for her own sexual health.

But perhaps Sylvia's doctor is right. The reason why we don't give new mothers ten sessions of vaginal rejuvenation is not because we don't care about a woman's health, but because it just sounds a little too sexy. Really, what would happen if every new mother in America received her own "electric dildo"? Do you suppose she'd start thinking about s-e-x?! Do you suppose she'd go out and buy some fancy lingerie? Do you suppose she'd experience *pleasure*?

Well, yes! And perhaps this is why we don't give new mothers (or any women, for that matter) their ten sessions. This is the great divide between life in France and life in America. Pleasure in France: good. Pleasure in America: naughty.

So, I wonder—is this the secret to *ooh la la*? Could it be as easy as getting a vaginal rejuvenation? I ponder all these questions as I walk down the stairs and out the door, and into the brilliant sunshine on my way to the Métro. This is where I see the Julia Roberts poster for the movie *Eat Pray Love*. It's late coming to France, but now here it is. There's Julia Roberts sitting on a park bench in Italy, savoring her gelato. She looks happy with the little plastic spoon poised between her lips, in love with the sensual creamy sweetness of her little treat. But there's something missing. I stand next to the poster for some moments and think. *Eat.* Yes, she's got the ice cream. She loves her ice cream, and Julia Roberts looks so sexy there in Italy. So we have *Love*. But *pray*? Pray? I recall the American poster for the movie—yes, in the American version, there's a nun sitting right next to Julia on that park bench outside a cathedral in Italy. You don't see much of the nun, but she, too, is eating gelato in the American version. So, I guess she's the "pray" part in all of this and we are meant to imagine that there's some spiritual redemption in eating gelato? Or maybe that's just my interpretation. Maybe I'd like a little spiritual redemption the next time I find a reason to buy some gelato, or even a pint of Ben & Jerry's.

Here's the point—there is no nun in the French movie poster for *Eat Pray Love*. What does this mean? I'm not sure. But I can't stop staring at Julia Roberts caught in this moment of gelato reverie, spoon stuck in her mouth, eyes drifting sideways, little ballet slippers turned slightly inward giving her this air of innocence in the midst of all that pleasure—

and there's no nun watching her! There's no redemption. Just pleasure!

If you ask me, this is one of the big differences between American culture and French culture. We have a nun watching us while we take pleasure. I think we feel a need to struggle a little bit or at least get some kind of spiritual or physical or emotional benefit from our pleasure taking. We can't just have pleasure for the sake of pleasure. And so, in America, Julia Roberts needs a nun beside her to truly enjoy that gelato and remind her that she will have to pay for her sins. In France, it's all about the gelato and you don't need anyone looking over your shoulder, saying it's okay and that you should indulge every now and then, just as long as you pay for it later. And there's no one to say you deserve a break today. After all, you'll suffer for it—one way or another—sooner or later.

So, I wonder—is this part of the French secret to *ooh la la*? This lack of guilt? Recently, I sent an e-mail questionnaire to a group of French women. One of the questions was *what do you do when you feel guilty?* I was thinking about the guilt one feels from overeating or buying a pair of shoes that one cannot afford, or chasing after a boy that is really not worth one's time. Most of the French women just left this question blank, but one of them answered *guilty for what?*

As I understand it, this idea of guilt is foreign to French women. They don't tend to overindulge, and so they don't feel guilty. But here's what I think—it goes the other way around, too. They don't feel guilty, so they don't overindulge. And because they don't overindulge, they don't feel guilty.

So what if we all decided to let go of the guilt? Suppose we decided to feel fine with how we are right now? Wouldn't that be revolutionary?

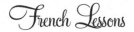

French Lessons

Find ways to take your pleasure, without guilt. You might want to start small. The quality is more important than the quantity. However, in order to really get into the practice of being a sensuous woman, you'll want to bring this small pleasure into your life on a daily basis. So, you might choose a time of day where you'll indulge in something delicious and a little bit sexy. It might be a small gelato or a bubble bath or a nap or sneaking off to an afternoon matinee. It should be something that on first blush seems a little naughty. But just a little naughty.

But first, do a little research. Find out what truly gives you pleasure. After all, gelato isn't on every woman's top ten list of indulgences. But still, it's important to think about what brings you a feeling of delicious sensuality. We live in a country that rewards those of us who work hard and struggle and suffer. Unfortunately, this can backfire when we feel as if we've had no real relaxation or joy, and then we go to the other extreme and overindulge. And next comes guilt.

So promise yourself a bit of pleasure every day. Find out what makes you feel as if you've treated yourself very well indeed.

Finally, take good care of the inside of your body as well as the outside. You might consider asking your doctor what you can do to tighten those pelvic muscles. Find out if certain yoga poses will help. And while you may not have vaginal rejuvenation treatments and electric biofeedback equipment available to you, I think your husband might be quite willing to assist in your quest for pleasure and ooh la la.

CHAPTER SIX

My Dinner with Coco

Charisma is the liberty to be yourself.
—MICHELINE TANGUY

IT'S EVENING IN PARIS, and I am on my way to meet the famous Coco. I am very excited about this because I have heard so much about her. In fact, according to my American friend Melanie, Coco has a whole lot of *ooh la la*! And Melanie should know. She was once married to Peter, who is now married to Coco. Still, she has a certain admiration for her ex-husband's French wife. *Oh, you've just got to meet Coco!* She tells me on the phone. *She's the quintessential French woman. She's always dressed up, always wears a scarf! You've got to meet her when you're in Paris. I'll set it up.*

And now, here I am in Paris. I clutch my little gift box of chocolates and hurry down the Faubourg Saint Honore to Peter and Coco's home. It's a gorgeous night, the sky is clear, and the weather has turned warm once again.

I pull on a big brass handle and open an enormous door that leads me inside the ancient building, and then I walk

through the courtyard, where I locate the elevator and up I
go. Peter answers the door. He is a handsome man in his
middle years. Well dressed. Well groomed. And this is not sur-
prising when I learn that for many years he wrote for *Vogue
Hommes* (Vogue Men). He ushers me into the apartment,
and I take a deep breath. The place looks something like a
movie set. A very romantic movie set—as if there is a delicious seduction about to take place. The rooms are awash in
deep mauve and red. In fact, one entire wall is painted red.
There are lots of silk pillows in hot pink, and mirrors and
little lamps with shades decorated with dangling crystal
teardrops. Oh, and there's music playing. Sultry jazz. And something in the oven smells very good indeed. Spicy. Peter tells
me he is making a standing rib roast.

So how are you enjoying your visit to our fine city?
Peter asks.

And I tell him I am having a wonderful time. I don't ask
him where his wife is, because I don't want to sound nervous. But for a fraction of a second my brain takes flight and
I imagine that I have landed in Morocco via the River Seine
and I am about to be seduced by a sultan. On top of this,
Peter is undeniably charming, welcoming me into the living
room, sweeping off my jacket, and disappearing with it and
then suddenly reappearing. He is talking a million miles an
hour, and while he tells me that Coco, her sister, Isabelle,
and their mother will be along shortly, he stations himself
behind the bar—and pops the cork on a bottle of cold champagne. He fills a flute, waits for the froth to settle, and then
hands it to me. He pours a glass for himself and motions for
me to try a *nibbly* and then passes a little dish of the most
thinly sliced salami I have ever seen.

Oh, and there are olives, too. Very French. Peter switches seamlessly from English to French to Paris to Cape Cod to Maine to New York City and back to Paris, where he tempts me with the expectation of finally meeting Coco. *Oh, you are in for a treat,* he tells me. And I am glad for this because it means she's really on her way, but still more time passes and she has not arrived. *Coco is fabulous. She is so French!*

He brings his glass up for a toast, clinks glasses with mine, and says, *a vos amours* (to your loves). I smile and think of my husband, Bill, far away in Australia.

I sip champagne and laugh at Peter's banter. For a moment, I imagine Coco walking in the door. What will she think when she sees me at the bar stool, legs crossed, drinking champagne and sharing *bon mots* about French lingerie with her American husband? This thought makes me a bit anxious. After all, I've heard she's a bit unpredictable. Perhaps even explosive. Suppose she doesn't like the looks of the friendly scene between her husband and a strange woman and she misunderstands my writerly intentions and then she screams something in French to me—something I don't understand? And then, suppose she grabs me by the hair and pulls me down on the floor and I break the champagne flute? And well, this is what I'm thinking when the door opens and Coco appears in a flurry of packages and perfume, accompanied by her sister Isabelle and mother and lots of *bisou bisou*, kisses all around. She greets me with a bisou on each cheek. My French is stuttering along at about twenty-five miles per hour and her French is zipping along at three hundred kilometers per hour. *Enchantée!* (which means nice to meet you, but sounds more like enchanted). And indeed, I am.

Coco is wearing a perfectly fitted tailored jacket, a pencil skirt, high heels, and as she talks—explaining how work was wild today and the judge in chambers said this and that— she click-click-clicks about the apartment. She takes off her jacket. I can tell she has said something funny about her day to Peter, but I'm not quite sure what. Coco and Isabelle are both attorneys. Apparently, they have their own private prac- tices, but they share offices and secretaries. After work, the two sisters met up with their mother and then they shopped for dinner. Coco goes into the kitchen and checks the roast in the oven and then she is cooing at Peter for being such a fabulous chef. *I love you, mon mari!* (my husband), she calls out, throwing air kisses from the kitchen.

There is the sound of water in a pot and the refrigerator opening and closing and packages being unwrapped and dishes being placed on the counter, and before I know it, the table is set, the candles are lit, and we are seated before dishes of food—the rib roast, now in delicate slices, a bowl of *haricot vert* (green beans), and new potatoes.

Coco holds court, gesticulating and laughing and just as quickly frowning in a way that is both scary and seductive. Peter sits back in awe of the powerhouse that is his wife. I do, too. And the meal goes on. There is red wine and white wine and then a salad course and more wine—this time a *digestif*, along with the cheese course. Ah, the cheese. It's like nothing I've ever tasted. So smooth and flavorful, even slightly lemony. Coco, Isabelle, and their mother tell me about the little farm they own in the south where they have goats and make and sell their own cheese. Yes, this magnificently creamy and tangy chevre is their very own. This woman who is a high-powered attorney, a woman with opinions on every- thing, so fashionable and sexy in her skirt and boots and cashmere sweater, makes her own cheese!

We are not from Paris, Coco explains. *We come from a little town called Saint-Julien-sur-Cher.*

Peter explains, *Coco's family has an organic farm there. This cheese you're eating—it's from the family farm.*

I tell her it's delicious.

It's called Selles-sur-Cher, Coco explains. *Our family has seventy-five cattle, forty goats, and chickens!*

Beaucoup de chickens, Peter adds.

We are country girls! Coco announces while slicing a bit more cheese and laughing.

I decide right then and there that it must be the secret to her *ooh la la.* She is funny and loud and completely herself. She is absolutely nothing like the stereotypical French woman. And yet, in a way she is. Because she's elusive. You can't categorize her at all. She's unique. And loud and fun besides!

And Coco and her sister and mother love to eat! This is not the typical image of the French woman—eating very little and having a cigarette for dessert. No, we are now having our apple tart tatin, even though I protest that I can't possibly eat anything else. But before I know it, the pastry is sliced and served on an elegant little plate. And then, the conversation begins to wind down. We sip our espresso, and Peter, who has let his wife take center stage all evening, quietly brings his guitar to the table and begins to play a song softly. I recognize it as Leonard Cohen's "Hallelujah." Yes, hallelujah, indeed.

What a night!

Later on in the taxi back to another French friend's home where I'm staying, I take this time to think. My friend Isabelle actually calls this moment her Secret Garden—the spaces in the day where you can stare out the window and just dream and think and relax. She says it's important not to miss these moments by throwing in some other activity, such as checking your iPhone, which I would probably be doing right now, if I had an international phone. But here I am, traveling through France with no phone at all, and so, I have a Secret Garden moment.

I think about Coco. She really doesn't fit into the mold of the ideal French woman. She's so friendly and bold. Yet, she's extremely French in that she's very fascinating and intriguing. And while she is not beautiful in the way American movie stars are beautiful and she's not terribly slender—I do believe it's her confidence and sense of self-possession that make her very beautiful and downright dazzling. It's her passion and zest for life. And her husband clearly adores her for all this and more. She's so complicated!

Anyway, this is what I am thinking as my taxi makes a right on Boulevard Saint Germaine and inches its way through the narrow side streets, which by the way are still filled with *Parisiennes*, click-clacking down the sidewalks.

It seems to me that whenever I am here—and not just Paris, but in all the small cities and villages of France—I am given a different message than the message I receive in my own country. And that message is—*you* are *good enough*. In fact, it seems to me that all of France is one big fan club devoted to the *Female*. And not just eighteen-year-old females, but older women as well. In America, I often feel admonished for my shortcomings. In France, rather than admonished, I feel encouraged to take better care of myself, and to dress well, to eat well, and to take pleasure wherever I can find it. Because, I'm a Woman! *Viva la différence!*

I don't think it's simply living in France or being French that gives these women their sense of beauty and mystery, because I have found more than a few women in my own country and other countries around the world that possess this special something, that mystery and confidence and *ooh la la.*

Yet it does feel to me that France is the epicenter of *ooh la la.* Or maybe it's just my *ooh la la.* I am still searching. But I do believe there's something in the air I breathe here that shifts my molecules and makes me want to be a better woman.

As I step out of the taxicab, I feel a few drops of rain hit my face and I am fortunate enough to tuck inside just before the downpour.

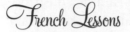

French Lessons

Host a dinner party. It doesn't have to be a major affair. And you don't have to make your own cheese, like Coco. You could make a roast, boil some vegetables, and then buy a few items at the store. Pick up a sweet at your local bakery. The point is that for a woman it's important to have an audience of sorts to build up your sense of fun and frivolity. Every day can't be a workday, and by adding some fun into your life you will soon discover your own unique gifts for entertaining, conversation, and maybe even music!

Finally, cultivate your Secret Garden. Put away your iPhone and embrace those found moments in your life, when you are alone and quiet and you really have nothing to do but stare out a window. These are just as important to your psyche as the times you spend laughing and entertaining. This is because, as women, we need a little mirror held up to ourselves to appreciate our own true beauty. And so, when you enjoy the company of others and they enjoy yours, you can see your own charms reflected in their eyes. We are made to be part of the larger world. And a dinner party is a simple way to join in on the theater of life.

!!!

CHAPTER SEVEN

I Am a Camera

Fashion is not something that exists in dresses only. Fashion
is in the sky, in the street, fashion has to do with ideas,
the way we live, what is happening.

—COCO CHANEL

IT'S THE NEXT DAY and the rain has just stopped. The sun is
shining all over Paris. Nonetheless, the streets are slick and
full of puddles, and since it is my last day before I leave for
the north, I decide I will get a "brush out." A shampoo and
blow-dry. And so, when I see a nice-looking hair salon off
Boulevard St. Germaine, I walk in and ask the pretty young
girl at the desk if someone can see me without an appointment. She says absolutely, and she introduces me to Benjamin, a stylish young man with blond highlights in his light
brown hair. Benjamin ushers me down the corridor and into
a private area where I find a smock. He takes me to the sink
and shampoos my hair. He asks me if it's still raining outside. I tell him no, that it's stopped, and before long we are
deep into a conversation about rain boots and fashion, and
I am so pleased to say that my new hairdresser, Benjamin, is

a wealth of information, especially on how the popularity of *wellies* all began in France! He brings me a little dish of violet candies from Toulouse and then as he's drying my hair he tells me the story of wellies.

A few years ago, wellies (short for Wellingtons) burst onto the scene in America, popping up on rainy days in bouquets of brilliant colors and later dizzying designs. But before this happened, Benjamin tells me, they were just ordinary dark green rubber boots. Sturdy. Practical. Reliable. Forgettable.

Wellies started in England over a hundred years ago. They were waterproof walking boots that were named after the Duke of Wellington—excellent for gardening or stomping around in the mud, through the marshes, chasing after your purebred hunting dogs.

That was the story for decades until one day, Benjamin explains, *the beautiful French supermodel Inès de la Fressange was sighted walking down a Paris street. It was a rainy day and she was wearing her wellies!* The original, plain, dark green ones.

Where did she get this brilliant fashion idea? She probably saw people wearing them during a recent visit to England, but according to my hairdresser on the Left Bank, it was Inès who brought the most recent wellies craze to Paris and hence to the world. She, and she alone, is the one who set the streets abuzz wearing these strangely plain, but somehow compelling boots. They were so old, they looked new. They were an overlooked classic. And the next thing you know, the wellies craze quickly spread to the rest of France and then to the United States, and, well, probably all over the world. And even the English people began to see their wellies with new eyes.

The point is, he says, *in Paris, the fashion is born in the streets. It's recreation for people.* He pauses, takes the blow dryer away from my hair for a moment, and smiles thoughtfully as he directs the blow dryer toward his face, letting the warm air blow back his own bangs off his forehead. He smiles wistfully, taking his time. For a moment, I wonder if he's going to forget about my hair and begin styling his own. He looks at me through the mirror and then tries to focus on *moi.*

You know, he continues, *on the news in France, the journalists will talk about the fashion people. It's very special to Paris—the sport—to look at the people from the café. In London and the United States you don't have that. Here, we take these ordinary things like the boots and we turn them into something else. Sometimes it works. Sometimes it doesn't. But it's like this—we have Le Regard. That's very important.*

And then he goes back to drying my hair, coaxing a few curls with his fingers, and tells me that fashion journalists from all over the world come to Paris to see what will be the next big thing. Next thing you know, these street styles appear in the designers' new collections and filter down to the magazines and the movie stars.

What I love about this is the understanding that ordinary women can change fashion. Yes, special attention will be paid to someone like Inès de la Fressange, but if fashion truly begins on the street, then it is possible for any woman to have the power to influence the world, and what the world finds beautiful. It's just a matter of jumping into the conversation.

And fashion is a conversation. It's a conversation that's been going on since the first cavewoman decided to switch things up and wear her animal furs draped over one shoulder, sewn together with a needle made from bones, and then suddenly this look began to appear all over the savannah! The look makes a reappearance in the draping style tunics of ancient Greece, and again with Madame Grès in the 1930s, who stylized the look in matte silk, paying homage to classic Greek columns and architecture.

I love the scene in the film *The Devil Wears Prada* when Meryl Streep, playing the *Runway Magazine* editor-in-chief, gives her assistant a little history lesson on the journey of fashion:

I see. You think this has nothing to do with you. You go to your closet and you select . . . I don't know . . . that lumpy blue sweater, for instance, because you're trying to tell the world that you take yourself too seriously to care about what you put on your back. But what you don't know is that that sweater is not just blue, it's not turquoise. It's not lapis. It's actually cerulean. And you're also blithely unaware of the fact that in 2002, Oscar de la Renta did a collection of cerulean gowns. And then I think it was Yves Saint Laurent . . . wasn't it who showed cerulean military jackets? I think we need a jacket here. And then cerulean quickly showed up in the collections of eight different designers. And then it, uh, filtered down through the department stores and then trickled on down into some tragic Casual Corner where you, no doubt, fished it out of some clearance bin. However, that blue represents millions of dollars and countless jobs and it's sort of comical how you think that you've made a choice that exempts you from the fashion industry when, in fact, you're wearing the sweater that was selected for you by the people in this room from a pile of stuff.

* * *

But now, I would like to take this notion of fashion's influence one step further. Let's imagine that the magazine assistant then takes her blue sweater home, and the next day, she decides to wear it backward or inside out or she cuts out some heart-shaped holes down the sleeves? Or suppose she pairs it with an unlikely black pencil skirt and her grandmother's green cloche hat. She is channeling an old film she saw. She is inspired by Louise Brooks. And she wears her ensemble, walking down the street and then The Sartorialist snaps her picture or Bill Cunningham jumps off his bike and gets his camera out and then she appears in *The New York Times* Sunday Styles section. Or perhaps it's her best friend who's studying photography at the San Francisco Art Institute and she decides to photograph her friend in her ensemble and then she posts a picture of her on her Facebook page and then another friend does a blog about her and her unique look? Just consider the fourteen-year-old Tavi's *Style Rookie* blog or the photos of gorgeous eighty-year-olds featured in the blog, *Advanced Style*.

The point is—this is how fashion conversations begin and this is how trends are made. Yes, the fashion designers will pick up on it and yes, it will filter down to your local Casual Corner, but it begins with you and your own imagination.

Back on the Left Bank, I say my *au revoirs* to my hairdresser, Benjamin, and walk out onto the street. It's a brilliant day, sunny and just a little cool. There is hardly any sign that it ever rained, and somehow my eyes have been refreshed by my conversation in the salon. I look at all the French women—and the men, too—a little differently. The man in the slightly rumpled raincoat standing in front of the magazine kiosk reminds me of my father in his commuting days in the 1960s on the New Haven Railroad.The lady cross- ing the boulevard wearing a blue scarf on her head makes me think of my grandmother and how she protected her fresh coif with a silk scarf tied neatly at her chin. When I see a twenty-something stand before me at the Métro Cluny La Sorbonne, I cannot help stopping and staring at her red plaid skirt. It's short and pleated, but it echoes back to all those Catholic schoolgirl skirts I remember watching from the point of view of a public schoolgirl spying on another world.While it is a MacLennan plaid, made famous many moons ago in Scotland, it has traveled far and wide down the cor- ridors of private schools to Punk artists to Grudge to the posters on the Champs-Elysées advertising the *reentrée* (back to school) with pretty girls wearing kilts and cozying up to a Scotsman playing the bagpipes.

Oh, yes, it's traveled even to me—a *femme d'un certain âge* who still keeps her lucky red plaid skirt in the closet and wears it occasionally (yes, the zipper doesn't always quite go up, but still—it kind of fits!). All this because I met the man who would become my second husband when I was wearing that red plaid skirt.And for a moment, before the burst of wind from the oncoming train rushes through the tunnel and separates us, I have a secret, silent conversation with the French girl in the red plaid skirt and I whisper to her in French and in English that she is a part of my story and I am a part of her story. And one day, when I am gone from this world, it will be okay because there will still be girls wearing red plaid skirts meeting the man of their dreams.

The next day, I am waiting at the train station, on my way from Paris to Lille in the north. I'm a little early and I have

about an hour and a half to wait at the Gare du Montpar-
nasse before the train arrives. And so I stop at the little
boulangerie in the station and buy a sandwich for the ride.
The French don't seem to make sandwiches with the flat,
square bread, like we do in America, but rather they manage
to fit some chicken, mayonnaise, and lettuce into a mini baguette, and it's delicious, plus it's so crunchy and chewy it's
impossible to wolf down. You must take your time and enjoy
every morsel.

I pay for the sandwich, along with a bottle of Evian. Then
I stop at the book kiosk and buy a copy of *French Glamour*, which is very different from the American version. It's
smaller and full of practical little fashion and beauty tips. I
save it for the train, because while I'm waiting in the station, I like to practice *Le Regard*, the art of looking. I situ-
ate myself on a bench where I can see the big clock in the
center and the huge black board that flips every so often to
show the arrivals, departures, and gates. And this is when I
spy a girl coming up from across the station, walking toward
the clock. She is wearing red ballet shoes, skinny jeans, a
ponytail, and a blue and white–striped French sailor shirt.
Oh, and a red scarf, wrapped around her neck several times
over, forming a little cocoon and breaking up the lines of
the stripes. Somehow, I find the sight of her in that striped
shirt absolutely mesmerizing.

I've always loved sailor shirts. This is probably because
they carry so much history. French sailors wore them hundreds of years ago when it was part of their official uniform;
then Picasso made them famous. There's a great old photo
of him, facing a window, the panes forming a kind of prison,
as he stares out with a distinct look of artistic frustration.

The blue period is not yet blue. Perhaps it's more of a purple, and he is struggling with his vision. Then again, it could
be simply that his newest mistress, Françoise, was a little
cranky that day. But it's the sweater that really gets me. I
know this sweater so well. It's certainly an iconic shirt, and
Picasso was just one in a long line of people to wear them.
Marilyn Monroe wore one on the beach. Brigitte Bardot wore
one while posing in red capris with red ballet flats on a red
sports car. Coco Chanel wore hers with wide-legged trousers.
Jean Seberg wore one with a pixie cut in the Jean-Luc Go-
dard film *Breathless.*

And I wore one. Actually, I still do. I started this obsession
with striped shirts when I was ten years old, and I believe
it was some kind of homage to the Beach Boys. Still, the
striped sailor shirt I really remember was the one I wore
when I was twenty-one. I bought mine in Paris and had returned to London, where I met Brigitte Roth. That's the girl
who bought me my first tube of red lipstick from Marks &
Spencer. She had been in London for a whole year, so she
knew all the places to shop—like Biba and the Kensington
Flea Market. Brigitte was from Vienna on a fellowship to study
fashion and theatre photography at the London design school,
Central Saint Martins. She had a big influence on me because
she was a few years older, and so stylish and original. Yes,
she wore bright red lipstick, but she also painted sparkles
on her government-issued prescription eyeglasses, and she
introduced me to vintage. We would spend Saturdays scour-
ing the flea markets in Kensington and Portobello Road. She
had Siamese cat-like blue eyes and reminded me of Marlene
Dietrich.

Brigitte and I lived in a flat in Highgate with an international bunch of twenty-somethings—a girl from Greece, who told me about the available room in the first place—another girl from France, who was hardly there because she stayed mostly with her boyfriend; oh, and there was one boy from Australia and another girl from Canada. But it was Brigitte and I who really bonded. Georgia, the girl from Greece, warned me that Brigitte was "very messy." And so, I was a little nervous the first time I walked into her bedroom.

And truthfully, it was the most gorgeous mess I have ever seen! Every single wall space was covered in photographs and magazine clippings and quotations, and it was so mesmerizing. I felt as if I had been swooped up and sent to a museum of fashion and beauty. There were women with crazy hairdos and photos from the 1940s, strange pictures of shoes, and pages torn from travel magazines with images of safaris and lions and elephants. There were clip-outs of little layer cakes that looked like hats. Honestly, I thought I could spend a year looking at these walls and I would still never grow tired.

Brigitte turned to me and said, *these are my inspiration walls*. And I just nodded my head, wordless. And then she asked me about posing for her. And whether I would dress up like a French girl—or how we both imagined a French girl would dress up—with my beret and my striped sailor shirt, with my very American Frye boots.

And I said, yes, of course!

That was just the beginning. I posed for lots of photography projects for her, and even today I have the photos framed on my walls. And these photos and memories are now all I have left, because I'm sad to say Brigitte had MS and she died quite young.

And now, you see, I can't look at a striped sailor shirt without thinking about Brigitte and remembering the times we had together.

Not too long ago, another good friend of mine passed away. Her name is Jackie and I miss her, too, every day. At her memorial service, Lloyd, another climate change scientist who works with my husband at Woods Hole Oceanographic Institute, arrived wearing a blue and white–striped sailor shirt. Now, you might think this is odd for him to wear such a shirt on this occasion, but actually it was perfect for Jackie's memorial service. After all, Jackie was an artist, a graphic designer, and definitely a free spirit. I met her after she was already quite frail—from the effects of Parkinson's. She was only in her early forties, and even with her difficulties with speech and her wide-eyed stare, I found her beautiful. And charming. She made me laugh, and since I was a newcomer to a town that was so strange to me—filled mostly with scientists—this was no small thing.

And so, I told Lloyd that I quite liked his French sailor's shirt, and he said I was mistaken! It's a Russian sailor's shirt. I had to laugh, even at this moment of great sadness, because through my tears I could still see how passionate we all are about clothing and how this simple shirt represented the delicate threads between a friendship in London, a striped shirt, another friendship years later, and another striped shirt. How could I tell him that seeing this shirt—whether it was French or Russian or Japanese—gave me solace, that in a world where we lose such beauty and art every day, there is still a continuing story and we all have a part in this story called life, love, fashion, and friendship?

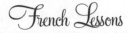

French Lessons

I know a lovely lady in America. Her name is Ruby and she has a blog called Ruby's Musings. I've never actually met Ruby, but I became friends with her because of her blog. It features lots of black-and-white photos of her sporting a Louise Brooks bob and flapper dresses and Capezio-style dance shoes. She posts all sorts of pictures of silent film heroines. This is what really captured my attention. I am a big fan of the fashions of the 1920s, and so when I look at her blog, I just feel happy. When I asked her about her style choices she told me that she discovered vintage as a child and often combines pieces in unexpected ways. She goes for a certain ladylike look that is not always easy to find, but through artful pairings, she creates wonderful looks. For inspiration, she looks at silent films, old photos, and listens to music from the 1920s and 1930s. Her look is charmingly romantic and nostalgic.

I am mentioning her here because she's a great example of how one jumps into the style conversation. You may think that you're idling away the day when you're looking at fashion blogs or watching interesting videos or renting the same kind of movie over and over again. You may assume this is a waste of time, but really, it's not. It's important work. And so is daydreaming about childhood memories and contemplating what kind of furniture or architecture moves you.

These obsessions are actually little clues to your style profile. Pay attention to what you are attracted to, because this is your "gold," your unique taste and a key to your own happiness.

Create a look book and use this to MapQuest your future self. This is what Ruby does. And actually, I have one, too. I have a big three-ring notebook filled with old family photos and pictures from magazines and catalogs that I've collected over the years. My good friend Jackie, a graphic artist, taught me to do this. And you know what? It's really helpful in honing in on one's dreams and visions. It's not just about fashion; it's about finding out who you are in this life.

!!!

CHAPTER EIGHT

~

These Boots Were Made for Walking

Without emotion, there is no beauty.
—DIANA VREELAND

I JUST DON'T buy this ooh la la business! Margie tells me this as she expertly shifts her little car into third gear. We are circling a roundabout just outside of Lille in the very northern part of France, on our way to her home way up by the Belgian border.

And what countryside it is! It's very flat and very green. So different from Paris, which now seems as if it belongs to another continent. This land where Margie lives just goes on forever and ever, far into the horizon. In fact, it's so flat, you might think you're in the Midwest, where Margie is originally from. Except here in northern France, the plains are dotted with old wooden windmills. Yes, *windmills*—because this part of France was originally a part of the Dutch Republic, that is, until 1673 when France invaded and conquered the country.

It's so interesting to me that my dear friend would ultimately find herself in a place where her Dutch ancestors might have been quite comfortable living. This is what I am thinking as I stare out the window, drinking in the scenery, the van Gogh yellows and the dark green moodiness of the land, dotted with golden haystacks.

Beautiful, I whisper, and Margie agrees, nodding, and she then picks up the conversation we began the moment we met up at the Lille Flandres train station two days ago. *And don't forget. France isn't Paris! Paris is New York and New York isn't America!*

Yes, but the French women. They're more romantic than American women, don't you think? And all those dinner parties. The perfume! The lingerie! Ooh la la!

She laughs at me and my crush on the French.

It is getting dark by the time we reach Margie's home. We park on the street across from a huge cathedral that is surrounded by a tall hedge. I catch sight of the cemetery with its crosses just peeking up above the green shrubbery. The sky is now a slate gray and Margie tells me it's going to rain tomorrow. We cross the street and Margie unlocks the big wooden door to her home. It was once a *charcuterie* and still has the feeling of a shop when you first walk in. The floors are made from the original tile work—blue and red and yellow, with little diamond shapes within circles. There is a big entryway where I imagine there were once chickens hanging in the big picture window and a French husband and wife stood by greeting their customers and swapping stories.

I tell Margie she should open up a shop here, but we can't decide exactly what kind of shop it should be. A school to teach English? She's known in town as the lady who speaks

English, and she actually once received a crank phone call from a little boy who blurted out in a thick French accent, *Hello! My name is English!*

Margie and I get settled in, and as she prepares dinner for the two of us, she tells me the story of how the children in the neighborhood got acquainted with her:

Part of it is that I decided a few years ago to do Halloween to endear myself to the local children—being very careful not to dress up as a witch because Morbecque is famous for witches (some were burned here in the Middle Ages, I believe) and I did not want anyone to think I might be one. This is why that little boy would be aware of me, because I answer the door "trick or treat!" and I speak English to give them a thrill.

However, I got sick of doing it—partly because the French kind of decide to do Halloween on the day that suits them (very *typical), not sticking to the 31st—and once when the 31st was an inconvenient day like a Monday, I was stuck with tons of candy so I said, okay, I'm not doing it anymore. (Plus when the kids do come in force they get older and older and they have no costumes at the end and they ring my doorbell really late—but I did throw up the window and shout out," 'alloween, c'est terminé!" [Halloween is over] and they got the message. And now there's a group of teenagers that are very polite to me and say* bonjour).

This year, on the way home on Halloween, about five p.m. (that I was not *going to observe), I stopped at the supermarket, and as I was coming out of the store and walking to my car, I heard a couple of little voices from boys on bicycles waaaaaaaaay far away from me (and several miles from my house I might add) and they were shout-*

ing at me, "Madaaaame, madaaame, Halloweeeeeeeeeeen, Hal-
loweeeeeen." *Damn. I went right back into the store and
bought about twenty euros' worth of candy, raced home,
and had a good turnout. So I guess I'm stuck with it.*

We laugh about this over dinner. Margie cooks a delicious
salmon with a salad and then we turn to our memories.
Margie and I met back in 1977 when we were both studying fiction writing at NYU. She was so tall and slender, she
really could have been a fashion model. She had an adorable
pixie haircut and was two years older than me and bursting
with talent. At the time, she was writing a novel about her
experiences in stand-up comedy. I found her fascinating. We
became very good friends and I asked her to be my brides-
maid. We've remained good friends through both our mar-
riages and our divorces and then for me, a new marriage.
But here's the thing that solidified my friendship with Margie.
On December 31, 1983, I was very, very pregnant—in fact
almost two weeks overdue. My midwife at the maternity center advised me that I would not be able to have my baby
with her, but that I would have to go to the hospital if I did
not go into labor by January 1. She advised I try taking castor oil. And so, on New Year's Eve, I did my best to go into
labor. I bought a bottle of castor oil and while my husband
and Margie drank champagne and celebrated the arrival of
1984, I took several tablespoons of the god-awful stuff.

But, you know what? Margie took a tablespoon, too. As a
form of sisterhood, she told me. And she agreed; it tasted god-
awful. And we laughed and laughed. And here it is, almost
thirty years later, and we are still laughing.

And so the evening goes, a long, luxurious dinner in her
kitchen with her cats curling up around her feet as the night

grows quiet and we are surrounded by the feeling that we have all the time in the world. I admire this sense of appreciation for ordinary moments, and it occurs to me that perhaps Margie is more French than she would like to admit. We sip our tea and she shows me to my room upstairs. Oh, but before that, she takes out her new raincoat. It's a very simple, very elegant black number with big black buttons and a poofy collar. Then Margie shows me her old raincoat, which is also very nice. It's made by a small Parisian designer, Et Dieu Créa la Femme—named after the Brigitte Bardot film *And God Created Woman.*

Margie suggests I try it on. And then she tells me that she would like to give it to me. *This is a very good French designer,* she says, and it does look nice on me. It's a little long, but not too long, and it has the most wonderful clasps— really delightful hardware—and a soft material that feels warm and comfortable. I love the coat, and it's not just the material. It's the fact that Margie wore this raincoat during many rainy days and it still contains her aura. If I take this raincoat home with me, I am taking a little bit of Margie with me. And so I say yes, I will take her raincoat. Oh, and I give her my little classic trench coat that I bought at Target, which she adores. So, we have had a bit of cross-cultural fashion exchange!

Here's the interesting thing about expats. They are not so enamored of the French. They say, *yes, yes, it's beautiful, and they love the wine and the food and the chic women, but just try to get your cable installed!* It's not easy being an expat. And I think it's not just that they see the cracks in *la vie en rose*, but when they visit America, they cannot help but compare it to France and they find America to be not up to par. And so, they return to France, where they miss America. *The convenience! The straightforwardness of the place! The Reese's mini peanut butter cups!*

Oh, and their American friends and family, of course.

And so, they are lost somewhere in the middle, never feeling quite at home. This isn't the case for all expats, I know, but for some, it is true.

It seems to me that there must be a way to combine the cultures. I know for me, I want to keep a little French and take it home with me. I want to go back twice a year and get my French fix. I want to learn from the French and reconnect with my own roots, but I want to be American. I do believe if I weren't American, I probably wouldn't find the French quite as fascinating as I do now. And if I were French, I would probably find the Americans incredibly fascinating. This is what a salesgirl at the Paris Sephora told me. *Ah, I love the accent Americaine! It is so pretty!*

The next day while Margie teaches at the university, I go shopping. I love shopping in Lille. In Paris, nothing seems to fit me, and I feel decidedly unchic, but in Lille I feel just right. All the big Paris stores are there, too—Galeries Lafayette, Printemps. And C&A, which is actually a German store; as well as Zara, which is Spanish; and H&M, which is Swedish. But never mind—the point is, I am shopping. Although, I actually don't buy much. This is to save money, but also because I am worried about my luggage. It's not easy to negotiate suitcases on trains and Métros and planes, so I try to limit myself. Mostly, I enjoy taking photographs of things I like—and so I dash in and out of stores, resisting the temptation to buy.

That is, until I come across a pair of red boots. I love red boots.

I've been thinking about red boots for a long, long time. First in 1978 when my boyfriend, the stand-up comic who would later become my husband and then my ex-husband, and I were traveling through Amsterdam. His friend, another American who had studied with him at the University of Kiel in Germany, met us at a café/bar. He said his girlfriend would be there shortly. We ordered Heinekens and the men began speaking in German—about old times, about how they met at Harpur College, about the sixties, and who knows what else. I really couldn't follow much, and so I entertained myself by staring out the window.

I discovered her before she even came through the door. Perhaps I fell a little in love with the girl with the long brown hair and the red boots. She swept into the bar and leaned down, kissing her boyfriend, on each cheek, introducing herself to us. She spoke quickly in English, switching to German, to French, and back to English. She was so happy, she said. She got a job writing for a newspaper! She was a journalist. I wanted to be a journalist, too, I told her. And then she looked at me and said, *it pays for shit you know. Merde!* And then she took a swig of her boyfriend's Heineken and went on, *excuse me, but I am really bummed out because I paid so much for these boots and look! Merde!* She bent down and took the red boot off her right foot and showed us how the heel was cracking. Both of the men quickly assured her that she was completely correct to be upset and that she should return them to the shop immediately. And I agreed. Yes, bring them right back to the shop! But in reality, I think they were mesmerized by this girl, her accent, the temper, her constant use of the word *merde*, and the red boots. I know I was! She was twenty-seven and I was twenty-four. She was French and I was American. And I decided I wanted to be her when I grew up.

The next time I thought about red boots was in Wimberley, Texas. I had just attended the AWP (Associated Writing Conference) in Austin, and after the conference, my friend Joel drove into Austin and picked me up so that I could visit with him and my good friend, mentor, and muse, Paula Martin. But before we drove up the mountain to their house in the hills, Joel and I stopped for lunch by the river. And right next to the restaurant, we found a vintage cowboy boot shop. I tried on a pair of red cowboy boots. They fit perfectly and more than this, they were the same cowboy boots that Meg Ryan wore into the office at Paramount (I was her assistant many years ago). She was wearing a flimsy flowered hippie dress, and she was just a little bit pregnant. Her hair was long because she had just finished filming *The Doors* movie. Still, it was the cowboy boots that I found mesmerizing. It took Meg's very soft, very feminine—almost fragile—look, and added this edge. Before that day, I never considered cowboy boots. I always imagined if you wore cowboy boots, you'd also have to wear jeans and a cowboy hat, and then you'd have to learn line dancing and bull riding, and well, you can see where my mind was going. No cowboy boots for me!

And then, all that changed.

The point is—we are all Meg Ryan. We are all that French girl with her broken heel in Amsterdam. Because whether you know it or not, you are inspiring someone. You are changing someone's life forever.

And so here in Lille, I pick up the red boots. They are actually not cowboy boots, but kind of an amalgam between ankle boots and cowboy boots. They do have those little tabs on each side. I ask the saleslady if she has them in my size. Luckily, the bottom of the boots lists the sizes for Europe, the U.K., Italy, and the United States. And so she goes to the back and brings back a box. She does not help me try them on, for which I am grateful. I get a little embarrassed when someone puts shoes on me. I'm not sure why. It just seems so awkward.

Anyway, these boots fit! These boots are made for walking! I love these boots. I walk up and down the length of the store, and all the salesladies agree. I definitely look good in these boots. I stare at my feet in the mirror and realize that these are better than Meg Ryan's cowboy boots. They're very cool and modern, and the color is so rich, kind of a cranberry red. And of course, I do have a thing for red.

I take my boots up to the cash register and tell the clerk that I would like to buy these boots. She is pleased by this, but then tells me that the boots will need *protección*. She says this in French. "Protection" in French is the same as it is in English. It's just that when someone says *pro-tech-shion* in French, it sounds a little ominous. Then again, that could be just me.

What do you mean? I ask her, and she explains that I cannot, absolutely cannot wear these boots in the rain or they will lose all their color. *You mean all the red will go?* I ask, and she nods gravely. *Oui.* And then she places a big canister on the counter. It's a can of "Shoe Beauty Balanced Care." It's written in English, because as it turns out the boots I am about to wear are from Sacha, a shoe company in the Netherlands, not French. So perhaps my boots are more like the French girl I met in Amsterdam, after all. I ask if she can't just spray it on right now and she says, no, that I must buy it. I explain that I cannot buy this can of "Shoe Beauty Balanced Care," because I will not be able to take it on the airplane with me, and besides I don't want to carry a big can of stuff with me back down to Paris and over to Normandy and then Rouen and the south, but I don't tell her this exactly, I just say, *ça va bien*. It's okay. I will manage without the Shoe Beauty Balanced Care. I will take my chances. I want the red boots.

The saleslady tentatively hands me the bag with a worried expression. *Vous comprenez? Sans protección!*

I take the bag and reassure her. *Je comprends. Sans protección.*

And so, I walk out of there with the red boots, but without protection.

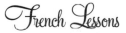

French Lessons

Beauty is about context. Consider this—a woolen beret looks chic and fun when you wear it in the United States. When you wear your adorable beret in Paris, your French friend will beg you to please take it off. It's just not cool. And it probably reminds her of that Chevy Chase movie, European Vacation. *The point is, a beret worn in France has no irony. It just tries too hard. But your beret in America? Fantastique!*

It's the same with clothes. Your raincoat may have lost its luster for you, but try switching with a friend. It's not only a way to bring new life to old clothes, but it's also a great way to edit and re-think your wardrobe.

Consider what your icons are. For me, it's the striped sailor shirt, but for you it might be a pair of brown and white saddle shoes, or a charm bracelet that belonged to your favorite aunt. Maybe it's that sweater your boyfriend wore in college—the one that he would loan you occasionally. Oh, let's be honest—it's the one you would temporarily steal from him because you loved the scent of him on it.

The point is, clothing has a language and a desire all its own. The next time you walk out the door in an ensemble that you put together, know that you are having a conversation that began many, many moons ago, and is still continuing to this day.

And finally, accept that there is no "protection" when it comes to red boots or human beings. We take our chances. We walk into the rain. We travel a long distance and we must be brave and hope for the best. But in the end, the future's not ours to see.

Que sera, sera.

!!!

CHAPTER NINE

~~~~~

French Women Don't Do Plastic

And the beauty of a woman, with passing years, only grows.

—AUDREY HEPBURN

I AM IN NANCY'S HOME—actually I'm in her kitchen. Nancy is getting her daughter, Lexie, ready to return to the afternoon session of school, giving the nanny a list and simultaneously reminding me that I need to stay on task. *When is this book going to get done!?*

Soon, soon, I say.

Chop! Chop! she says with a big smile and a little wink, as she pours a cup of coffee for me.

Nancy is tall and blond, with the bluest eyes you've ever seen. I should explain that Nancy is an American, but she's been living in France for the last thirty years—ever since she met and married a French man. A doctor. Whenever we meet up, I am always amazed at how different she looks from all the French women I see around France. In fact, in the context of Paris, Nancy looks almost as if she comes from Norway or Sweden rather than upstate New York. She's that blond. That slender.

Nancy and I met back in the 1980s at Estée Lauder, so we have known each other for a long time. She's about ten years younger than me, but she's much more businesslike and often reminds me that I need to stay on task. While we both met in Lauder's international sales promotion department—we ultimately ended up taking different paths. I took the artsy/writer route, while Nancy stayed in the cosmetic/skincare industry and at this point in her life is very, very successful. In fact, she's a vice president of marketing at StriVectin, one of the largest prestige skincare companies in the world. I'm here today to get her thoughts on beauty, skincare, perfume, *ooh la la*, and anything else she wants to tell me. And for the moment, she wants to tell me how to get my writing career in gear.

You should be writing a book a year. Get a move on! she says while making sure her youngest daughter has put on her Petit Bateau sweater for her walk back to school.

I must admit that this scene feels a little ironic to me, because I remember when Nancy was a wild child in her twenties. How she would stay out late after work and go out to the clubs, dancing and drinking White Russians, and occasionally go right from a night out, then back to work at Estée Lauder without ever having returned home. As for me, I was a young mother and so I rushed home at ten minutes after five each night to pick up my baby daughter and stop at the market to retrieve fixings for the night's dinner.

And now, thirty years later, here we are walking down the rue de Passy, with her young daughter between us. At the light we wait, and Nancy turns to me and says I must tell American women that they need to stop trying to look like young girls. *Listen, you've got to tell them that men are not turning their heads for the gals who have obviously had lots of work done.*

Well then, who are they turning their heads for? I ask. Truthfully, I already know the answer to this, but I just want to hear Nancy say it.

And she does.

The young girls! she tells me, giving me that look to say, I know what you're doing.

Still, I continue, *so, aren't American women just trying to look young?*

The light changes and Nancy holds tight to Lexie's hand as we cross. *Well, that's ridiculous and it isn't working!*

Well, what should they do—I mean, if they want to turn some heads? I ask. *What's the answer?* And in this moment, I know I really want to know, not just for my readers, but for myself.

And Nancy, as always, gives me a very straightforward answer: *Take care of your skin and act your age.*

Wow. That seems so straightforward.

We leave Lexie at her school and then return down the street, back to rue de Passy. Nancy takes me into the Marionnaud. This is a famous French perfumery chain that sells perfume, cosmetics, and body and skincare products. Nancy asks the beauty adviser about the sales for a particular Stri-Vectin product. She's always on the job. And then she explains to me the French woman's approach to beauty. *It's all about feeling sexy and good in their body,* she begins. *This is why they keep their figures, style their hair so it's natural, and wear high heels and lingerie.* And then Nancy, who is much more of a cute ballet flats, paired with some classic L.L.Bean, kind of gal, shakes her head and whispers, *The women here try to remain sexy until they are carted away!*

So, do they get face-lifts? I ask.

And at this Nancy is adamant. *No!* she tells me, and then adds that I must write how we women should support one another when it comes to growing older and having our faces change with time. *We should stop telling women they look terrific with all that Botox in their face because, honestly, we don't believe it. And we should stop reinforcing that looking young is the only way to look good. And lastly, someone should call out that men's heads only swivel for pretty young things and not for stretched, Botoxed, filler-filled older women.*

Wow. This is powerful stuff, but Nancy is in the business of skincare. She's lived in Paris for the last thirty years, so she knows what she's talking about.

We continue our conversation and browse the perfume department, and she tells me that French women will see their esthetician every three weeks for epilation or waxing. *They don't go in for manicures or pedicures. They like to take care of their nails themselves and they're not interested in a lot of high-maintenance treatments, but rather it's about the total look. So, no they don't do one extreme thing.* At this, she takes a sampler bottle of Estée Lauder's White Linen and spritzes it on one of the little cardboard sticks the store provides for testing. Nancy puts it under my nose and says, *remember those days!*

I take a whiff and laugh. *But, is it Estée Lauder?* I ask, putting on a serious face. And then Nancy laughs, because only someone who worked at Lauder in the 1980s would get this reference. Back then, every desk at Lauder had an eight-by-ten mirror framed in gold with an engraved question that asked, *Is it Estée Lauder?* This was meant to encourage the Lauder girls (and we were always Lauder girls, never women) to ask themselves when they're talking on the phone or filing fashion bulletins or writing the fall color story description for the latest *Tender Lip Tint* shades—*is it something that Mrs. Lauder herself would approve of? Would she chew gum? Never! Would she comb her hair at her desk? Absolument non!*

Now when I think back on it, I realize that we belonged to a very special sorority in a time when Mrs. Lauder still reigned supreme. And under her loving guidance, we were the ones to introduce the now iconic fragrance Beautiful to the international market.

Nancy puts the bottle back on the shelf and tells me, *you know for French women it's all about seduction. They want to be natural and accessible. That's why they won't do anything too extreme—whether it's perfume or makeup or crazy jewelry. They want to feel beautiful and that has nothing to do with a woman's age.*

Beautiful.

Just one word, but it means so much. There are so many instances where we use this word freely. Perhaps you said "beautiful" when you were just sitting on your deck with a glass of good wine in hand, witness to the last of the summer sunsets. It could have been the first time you looked into the face of your newborn baby. Then again, that feeling of awe could have come upon you when you were holding your dying mother's hand. She was gone to the world, but somehow her face was so tranquil and peaceful and finally free of pain that you thought, *ah, but she's beautiful.* In our hearts, we know that beauty has nothing to do with age or youth. It's about a feeling.

Certainly, France has no expiration date on beauty.

As American women, every day we are bombarded with images of youth and beauty, and the message is clear. Beauty is young. In fact, even to mention this is stating the obvious. But is it true? Recently, I picked up a copy of *French Vogue*. The entire issue was dedicated to the American designer Tom Ford, and it included his photographs of gorgeous *femmes d'un certain âge* wearing his designs. These women were not young, but yes, they were beautiful. And most of these women were not even French. We all know there are gorgeous French *femmes d'un certain âge*, such as Isabelle Adjani and Catherine Deneuve and Isabelle Huppert. But, here in *French Vogue* we had the American icon Lauren Hutton in a white jacket and white fedora with an impertinent feather tucked into the brim. Our American actress Marisa Berenson posed with her shoulder-length explosion of curls, wearing a blue sequin floor-length gown. The American artist and artist's muse, Rachel Feinstein, was also given the star treatment, her auburn hair complemented by crimson lipstick, nails, and an organza bolero that looked like something you'd order for dessert. And there was more—Ali McGraw in a white trench coat and Daphne Guinness in leopard. I had to ask myself, why do we never (or at least hardly ever) see these beautiful women in American fashion magazines—not just in advertisements for Talbots or rejuvenating creams—but the coveted high-fashion photo spreads?

In this one issue of *French Vogue*, I also discovered a series of absolutely shocking photographs by Tom Ford. Well, shocking to my American eyes. Yes, this was something you would never, ever see in a copy of *American Vogue* or *Elle* or *Glamour* or *Allure* or heaven-forbid *Self* (all magazines I love and adore). Here in *French Vogue* Tom Ford had eight full pages devoted to images of an older couple passionately kissing, touching, even groping! It was as if the camera had captured these very sexually charged moments in this couple's lives. The man and the woman in the photographs both had silver hair, lots and lots of wrinkles, and even age spots on their hands. They looked to be in their seventies, maybe older. And they were beautiful, not in spite of their age, but because of their age.

Tom Ford was quoted as saying, *Je suis fatigue par le culte de la jeunesse.* I am tired of the culture of the young.

Yes, and he's not alone. In France, you will see beautiful, stylish older women, not just in Paris and the major cities, but also in the little villages. They are sexy and they are revered. In fact, they are considered sexy because being older, and therefore wiser and more experienced, is very, very powerful and very, very alluring.

The question is—why isn't this true in America? Why do we equate youth, inexperience, lack of knowledge with beauty? It seems to me that what we need is a simple shift in our thinking.

We often see images of older men, wrinkled, gray, with gnarled hands and wizened faces, and we look to them as icons of male beauty. There is Clint Eastwood, Sean Connery, Harry Dean Stanton, Chris Cooper, and Harvey Keitel. These men are not exactly pretty to look at, certainly, but they are intriguing, classically handsome, fascinating, and powerful. You will often find them gracing the pages of *T, The New York Times'* men's styles magazine. Talk to a younger woman, say a twenty- or thirty-something-year-old, and she will tell you that they're "hot." Seems shocking, but this twenty-something is not simply responding to physical beauty. She is responding to the charisma of experience and accomplishment.

And this brings us to the question, why are we not as generous with women?

This is not a trivial issue, because if we live by the fountain of youth, then we will die by it. Think about it—this battle to stay as young looking as possible, no matter what our biological age may be—doesn't it send out a message to younger women that getting old, looking old, is horrible? And by saying it's horrible, we forfeit one of the great gifts of growing older—respect. The older male icons, by not hiding their age, occupy a place of honor in the national psyche that says—*yes, I've come this far, and have the lines and scars to show it*. As women, if we never look our true age, we will never earn this kind of respect. We will never become an "elder statesman" to our younger counterparts. This is a loss for us as women, and also for our daughters and granddaughters, who would love to look up to us but find this difficult and confusing when we act and look as if we are their contemporaries.

I adore the photographs of the artist Georgia O'Keeffe— especially the ones where she is in her eighties. She is wrinkled, for sure, but she is beautiful and completely herself. She's an inspiration, and I know many women who agree with me. So, why can't we be like that? A woman who is powerful and beautiful because of her age, not despite it.

That's authentic. That's real. And that's very French.

French Lessons

I love that Nancy said beauty has nothing to do with age, because I can think of so many moments when I found that something was beautiful because of its age. For instance, when I was in the market shopping for a vintage tablecloth, I came across a rusted wrought iron love seat. It needed some fixing. Some tender loving care. It definitely needed a new coat of paint. But, I thought, this is beautiful. I think a lot of us feel this way. We cherish the prospect of rescuing this treasure from the trash because we know the potential. We can see beyond all those scratches and chips and wear and tear to something extraordinary. Not extraordinary despite the scars of age, but because of them.

You see, when it comes to furniture or babies or sunsets or a delicious meal—we're very generous with the word beautiful. *And yet, with all this generosity of spirit, we are not always so generous with ourselves. In fact, we can be downright withholding and even un peu harsh when it comes to what we see in the mirror, especially past a certain age. Certainly, our American culture does not look kindly upon the older woman. The middle-aged woman. You see, in the United States, we don't even have a wonderful expression for a stylish, mysterious—dare I say, beautiful older woman. We must defer to the French who know the perfect expression,* la femme d'un certain âge. *The woman of a certain age. How mysterious, too!*

And it's true, in France, you will find many beautiful and confident femmes d'un certain âge, *but is this because they're not naturally better looking than American women or is this simply because they have more confidence and believe that they are beautiful, no matter what their age may be? I believe it's the latter. And that's good news for American women because it means that with a little emotional and intellectual "makeover," we, too, can feel beautiful in that mysterious French way—not despite our age, but because of our age. And yes, this internal makeover may involve an external makeover as well, but the key to beauty à la française is to begin with a complete understanding and acceptance of oneself. The French approach to beauty begins with knowledge—not simply knowledge about the world, but knowledge of your place in the world. Self-knowledge. From this vantage point, we can build our confidence and sense of well-being. We can be generous with ourselves and love ourselves. This just happens to be one of the French woman's most important secrets. And now, it's yours.*

!!!

CHAPTER TEN

The Scent of a Woman

A woman's perfume tells more about her than her
handwriting.

—CHRISTIAN DIOR

NANCY AND I LEAVE the store and walk out onto the street. She
has to go now because she needs to get back to work, but
before this, Nancy gives me a quick primer in the history of
the French *parfumerie*. The parfumerie culture is specific to
France, and we simply don't have the equivalent in America.
It's a place where you go specifically to choose a fragrance.

The traditional parfumeries are dying out, Nancy tells
me. *The femme de certain âge still goes, but the introduc-
tion of Sephora has changed everything. It's actually a French
company. And, it's revolutionary for America.*

*The younger women go there. It's all about what's new.
They're not looking for the latest cream. The pharmacie is
for older women. They'll buy all the creams at the pharmacie. The parfumerie is just selling the major beauty
products: Chanel, Dior, Givenchy, Clarins.* I should interject
that the French *pharmacie* is nothing like our CVS or Rite

Aid. It's a place where they sell specialized creams and beauty products and there's a pharmacist for medicine, who will meet with you in a private little cubicle and listen to you describe your ailments and then prescribe a particular medicine for you. You don't have to have a script from your doctor, because the French pharmacists have the authority to prescribe medicines.

Nancy continues her French beauty lessons. *French women,* she tells me, *are not experimental in their beauty regime. They stick to big brands and they're loyal to their brands and not looking to switch.*

I ask her if that's really true that French women don't do plastic, and she does admit that there are a few French women who may get a little face-lift when they're over fifty-five. *Never younger,* she insists. *And it's very, very subtle. They're more into cellulite creams and the waters for anti-stress. Everyone goes after you have a baby. You go for an entire week, even if you're not rich. It's to detox. There's no working out, no exercise. You sit around all day in a bathrobe and get baths with algae, and then you get hosed down.*

Wow, I think. Sign me up. I could really use a detox week at a spa!

Before Nancy and I say our *au revoirs* she insists that I go into one of the traditional parfumeries on the rue de Passy. I promise I will and then we kiss good-bye and I watch her walk quickly down the street, already feeling a little sad that our mini–Lauder Sorority reunion has come to an end.

And so, as promised, I walk farther down rue de Passy and I find a parfumerie. I open the door and a little bell rings, and here I am, in the world of French fragrance! *Secrets des femmes.* (Secrets of the women.) And what a world it is!

First of all, the place is empty. Well, not empty, exactly. There's a woman of an indeterminate age standing behind a long wooden counter. Her black hair is pulled back in a neat chignon and she's wearing a white jacket. It reminds me of a lab coat. Oh, and she has bright red lipstick on. The moment I walk in, she nods her head slightly and whispers, *Bonjour, Madame.*

And I whisper, *Bonjour, Madame* to her. And then we are silent. The place is so quiet that for a moment I wonder if the sounds of our voices will bounce against the ceilings and echo back. But actually, there is a lot of glass to absorb the sound. In fact, behind the counter, there are shelves and shelves of bottles of perfume. I recognize a few brands—the iconic Chanel No. 5; the new fragrance, Daisy, from Marc Jacobs with the flower top; and of course, there is Miss Dior's Cherie. And then there are lots of other fragrances I don't recognize. And truthfully, I am feeling rather intimidated. But the parfumer asks me if she can help me and so I simply say, I'm interested in the Miss Dior. She takes the bottle from the shelf and then sprays a bit on a card and hands it to me to smell. I should tell you this card is quite lovely. It's pink and folds up like a little gift with a bow. Inside, there's a photograph of Natalie Portman holding the bottle up to her lips, looking dreamily into some unforeseen future. I bring the card to my nose and inhale. And I will be honest here— it's not for me. I immediately know this. It's not just the patchouli scent that I recognize, but there is something much too young about this fragrance for me. Honestly. And it's not because Natalie Portman wears it. I tell the parfumer it's not right for me, and then she smiles slightly and shakes her head as if to say, I knew it. I could have told you that. We get into a little chitchat about life and travel and Paris and perfume. I tell her I'm a writer and I want to learn more about perfume.

And then she brings out a bottle that she has chosen just for me. Oh, and it's a gorgeous bottle. It's got a silver cover on the glass that looks kind of like a saddle. You flip this over to reveal the atomizer. *This is Voyage d'Hermès.*

Ah, Voyage! I'm a voyager. This will suit me. And I quickly spritz a bit on and start to rub my two wrists together, but the parfumer stops me, looking somewhat shocked, and says, *Non!* I ask why not and then she explains to me that this destroys the molecules. *You will scratch the notes*, she tells me, *chemically speaking.* And then she demonstrates the correct way to apply the perfume. She spritzes it into the air. *This way you let the alcohol evaporate.* And because she can see I am very interested in all these details, she continues by explaining the olfactory pyramid to me. *A fragrance has three levels of notes. The top, the middle—or la coeur (the heart), and then there are the bottom notes.* She spritzes the perfume into the air again and asks me to smell. *You see, the top notes are the notes that you can smell as soon as it's sprayed, the heart notes you smell after, and the bottom are the ones that remain on your skin after a few hours. They're the more obvious.*

I feel the fragrance as the gentle spray falls onto my face.

I like this fragrance. It's very lemony. In fact, it kind of reminds me of drinking my grandmother's iced tea (which was more like a combination of lemonade and iced tea). I can also smell freshly mowed grass, although I'm sure that's my imagination.

The parfumer explains to me that a fragrance lives on the skin and that this is why it will not smell the same on every woman. It all depends on chemistry. This fragrance is very different from the Dior, and I like it because it's not too flowery. And in fact, the parfumer tells me that both men and women wear Voyage d'Hermès. Still, I'm not sure I want a perfume that's so androgynous.

And this is when I see that choosing a fragrance is a lot more complicated than just deciding what smells nice and then going for it.

This is what my friend Vanessa has told me. She's from Paris, but these days she lives in Quebec. She's a marketing manager for Lise Watier, the biggest cosmetic and fragrance company in Canada. I met Vanessa through Jessica Lee—if you recall, she's my wonderful friend and traveling companion featured in *French Women Don't Sleep Alone*. The three of us (along with a couple of husbands and boyfriends and a few other French girls) met up recently at Cocagne, a French restaurant in the Plateau Mont Royal area of Montreal. Vanessa is very intriguing and very beautiful. We immediately began talking about beauty and fragrance. Oh, and here's a fun fact: Neiges, which means "snow," is the number one fragrance in Montreal and one of the top five in Canada. And I'd never heard of it! It's a Lise Watier fragrance. Still, I love the idea that the Canadians are wearing a fragrance called "Snow" because it truly speaks to the idea that a fragrance can reveal who you are and what you dream of and how very personal the choice is for each woman. Vanessa tells me that every fragrance can take a woman to a universe in her imagination. Sometimes she will choose it because it reminds her of a period in her life, a place, or a special person. It's connected to how you feel and how you want to feel and how you want to be perceived.

Later, I interviewed Vanessa about her experience choosing a perfume as a young girl growing up in France, and this is what she told me:

My first fragrance was Courreges in Bleu. Made by Courreges. I will always remember I went with my mom to a parfumerie. Sephora didn't exist back then and I went with her, and a beauty adviser had me smell. I was thirteen and I wanted something fresh and light. Not overbearing. It was like a ritual. Oh, my God, I thought, I'm entering this woman's world. The world of designer perfume. At that time, we were living in Boulogne. This was in the mid-eighties. My mother was wearing Nahema Perfume by Guerlain.

I remember how when we entered the parfumerie, you either knew what you wanted or you had to ask the beauty adviser and she took it out and sprayed. It was an entire ritual. My mom was into parfumerie and taking care of herself and I could feel I was entering this world of femininity, ritual, and secrets. My mother said to me, "Vanessa, you need to find a fragrance that corresponds with who you really are."

And standing here in Paris, a cloud of fragrance all around me, I realize the question at hand is not simply, what smells good to me, but who am I?

Really, *who am I?* And suddenly, I feel as if I am in a philosophical dialogue between Plato and Socrates and this beauty adviser is not only an expert on the olfactory pyramid, but the wisdom of self-knowledge. Truthfully, this is deep stuff.

Nancy and I were friends with another Lauder gal back in the 1980s. Her name is Debra Davis, and in fact, I'm still very good friends with Debra. She went on to open up her own public relations firm, but she's often said that she should have been a "nose." This is one of the highly trained professionals who actually create new fragrances. But there's the interesting thing about Debra. She was married when she was at Lauder. Both she and her husband were gay, but nobody really knew it. They had met in the 1970s and they had a marriage of convenience. Deb would wear Kate Hepburn-style clothes—wide leg trousers and turtlenecks. She favored simple tailored outfits because her wild mane of thick curly hair was her most eye-catching feature. She hardly wore any makeup, but since we all received freebies, she used to boast about using "buckets" of Estée Lauder's Night Repair. She recently told me the story of how she and her husband went to Spain to attend a cousin's wedding, and though all the young people knew that she and Mark weren't a traditional couple, the older people had no idea. At the wedding she met a girl from a very wealthy Spanish family and she learned that this girl and her sisters were wearing Eau Savage from Christian Dior. A man's fragrance! This was an awakening. And for Deb, wearing Eau Savage was the beginning of finding her true self.

So, this is how powerful and inspirational a fragrance can be. And perhaps this is why I have never been able to choose one.

Yes, despite the fact that I worked for a major perfume company for so many years, I have never been the kind of gal who wears fragrance.

When I was younger, I was really an Ivory soap kind of gal. You know, pure and fresh and clean. The idea of fragrance seemed so—I don't know—old-fashioned. And I thought of my mother and her Chanel No. 5 and how she left it on her bureau for so long, it went bad. Only I didn't know it had gone bad. I was only five years old and I picked up the half-filled bottle and sprayed it all over my neck, arms, and chest.

And boy, did it stink. But, I thought—this is what grown-up ladies do. This is something I'll just have to get used to.

And then by the time I was really ready to wear perfume, no one was wearing perfume. This was at the dawn of the 1970s and it wasn't cool. It wasn't something a good feminist indulged in. There were too many marches and rallies to fool around with such fripperies!

However, I did enjoy those shampoos that were filled with fragrance. Herbal Essences. I imagined that I was that girl on the commercial, shampooing my hair in the jungle. Naked under an enormous palm frond. Some parrots and monkeys cheeping in the background, admiring my lovely long honey-brown hair.

In those days, it seemed as if no one under thirty wore a fragrance—that was, until Charlie arrived on the scene. And then, suddenly it was okay to wear cologne. After all, Charlie was a career girl. She wore a sexy pantsuit and a hat and she was always in motion—taking big strides up the corporate ladder by day and being serenaded in jazz clubs by night. A little spritz of Charlie and she smelled great—not sticky sweet, but kind of kicky and cool and fun and a little like the way we imagined Annie Hall might smell. And I thought, if I wear Charlie then I will be the kind of girl to star in a Woody Allen film and everyone will think I'm hip and independent and artsy. But then we realized that Charlie was made by Revlon, and while we have only nice things to say about Revlon, the truth is every other girl and her younger sister can afford a Revlon perfume. We started to smell Charlie everywhere, and in fact, it started to become a kind of insult. *Oh, she wears Charlie!*

By this time, it's 1981 and everyone is wearing glitter and glossy lipstick and going to the disco. I was working temp at a law firm downtown, and I remember how impossible it was to get away from the smell of Opium. The cinnamon and orange undertones, the heady mix of incense and patchouli, overwhelmed me when I got in the elevator at the north tower at the World Trade Center. The building still felt new, and I remember how they were having trouble getting stores to open in the underground level. It was vast and confusing and a little like you'd entered the Land of Oz, but then everything in New York seems larger than life, bigger and better, and the heady mix of women with big hair and big shoulders and lots of perfume made me a little dizzy.

And then in 1984, I arrived at Estée Lauder and I met Nancy and Debra. They were younger than me and single, and so while they went out to glamorous clubs and wore Opium, I stayed home and watched from the sidelines. I wore Prescriptives Aromatique because it promised to soothe and calm, and as a young mother with a full-time job, that's exactly what I needed. During the day, I stared at my reflection in the mirror that asked me, insistently, *Is it Estée Lauder?* And by then, I could tell you if something was suitable for Estée Lauder, but I still couldn't tell if it was really me or not. And so, here I am, many years later, standing in a parfumerie in Paris inhaling the rose-infused, warm scent of Estée Lauder's Sensuous Nude. Yes, without my even mentioning the Lauder connection, she has chosen this for me. Truthfully, I'm a little embarrassed. Sensuous Nude? This seems a little naughty. This is definitely a grown woman's fragrance. I can't make up my mind—should I go with Voyage d'Hermès—and be the kind of woman who works as hard as Hemingway, travels around Europe with a little moleskin notebook, drinking at Harry's, when I'm not fishing and getting involved in the Spanish Civil War. No, perhaps I should be sensuous—

and nude—kind of like Collette—spending all day writing in bed with my papers and my fountain pen, eating chocolate bon bons and making love all night—that is, after performing a sexy pantomime act at the Moulin Rouge earlier in the evening.

And in that moment, I say yes. Yes, to Sensuous Nude. So what if I'm pretending? As I walk out of the shop with my little boutique bag, I think—I will grow into this. I may not be this woman now, but one day I will become the kind of woman who wears Sensuous Nude.

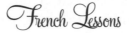

French Lessons

French women are taught to first find out who they are in this world. Yes, there are many, many fragrances to choose from, but a French girl is taught to decide first her essential self—and then she proceeds to find a perfume that matches her own unique personality, and style and intellect. As she matures and becomes a little more worldly, she might change her fragrance to something that is more complex and that can signify her experience, her travels, and her accomplishments. The French woman is in charge of the fragrance and not the other way around, and you can be, too, by simply asking for help and making a choice.

Be sure to take care of your fragrance by keeping it in a cool place like the fridge during the summer. Plus, it's very refreshing and this is what Marilyn Monroe did! Some French women will even keep their perfume in the box because it can be light sensitive.

Here's the wonderful thing about designer perfume. You

might not be able to afford a Chanel suit or a Kelly bag from Hermès, but you can borrow a little bit of that luxury by pampering yourself with the designer's fragrance. It's a simple and relatively inexpensive way to indulge in luxury. Many luxury bottles are refillable. And if not, they make lovely bud vases and look great on your dressing room table.

Finally, always spritz your perfume into the air after your shower or bath and walk into it. Don't spray it directly on your skin, but let the molecules fall all around your body.

!!/

CHAPTER ELEVEN

～

The Wisdom of the Femmes d'un Certain Âge

Elegance is not the prerogative of those who have just
escaped from adolescence, but of those who have
already taken possession of their future.

—COCO CHANEL

THANKS TO MY AMERICAN FRIEND, Deborah Krainin, I am being
introduced to a most fabulous French woman named Frédérique Duvignacq. Debby wants me to meet Frédérique because she is so stylish, unique, and adventurous. The two women
first met on holiday in Argentina. Debby was there for a few
years on a teaching fellowship and she decided to visit the
archipelagos of Chiloe. This is the little island where all the
penguins live. On her first day in Ancud, she met Frédérique
and Frédérique's partner, Pierre. They were both staying at
the same hostel. The owner of the hostel said they should
meet because they were all planning to go on the same expedition to the island. And so, they took the boat trip together and then they stuck together for the next week,

traveling each day to somewhere new in Chiloe, staying in different towns and enjoying each other's company every step of the way.

I do have to make one side comment here. This is a French girl, Frédérique—who is absolutely comfortable "sharing" her man with an American woman traveling on her own. All I have to say is *Vive la* sisterhood!

And so, Frédérique and I agree to meet in Paris at Café Le Fumoir. I take the Métro to Louvre Rivoli because it's such a beautiful day and I want to walk through the Jardin des Tuileries. I have plenty of time before our meeting and so I stroll past the fountains and statues of naked couples in warm embrace—and real couples, too—not naked, but yes, in warm embrace. They are tangled up together on the benches and the little metal chairs facing the fountains or on the green-green grass, inspired by the stone voluptuaries lining the park. And there are children, too—one little girl does a somersault, as if to entertain and delight one of the nearby stone nymphs.

I reach the Louvre and then leave the park through rue du Louvre and walk over to the rue de l'amiral.

And there, I meet up with Audrey Tatou. I mean, *Frédérique*—but really, she looks just like the famous French actress who stared in the film *Amelie*. This gal is so adorable and French and open and friendly and sweet that I feel as if I have just fallen into a story in a movie.

Of course, Frédérique—or as she prefers to be called, Freddie, is not aware of my girl crush. She simply smiles as we find a little table facing the street. She is wearing a simple gray top with a black sweater draped around her shoulders. Oh, and she seems to have hardly any makeup on and her lustrous brown hair is swept back into a casual ponytail.

Frédérique is wearing several strands of small, but very colorful wooden beads. They look like she might have bought them while visiting South America.

We exchange *bisous* (kisses) and we sit down and order a couple of glasses of mineral water. Frédérique tells me all about how she met Deb during the sabbatical year she took from her job. I'm amazed to hear that French companies not only allow but encourage you to do this, because it gives an employee an opportunity to take courses or travel or care for a new baby or elderly parent or to simply re-energize. And then, you can return to your job at the same salary. Frédérique is studying to enter the tourism industry. She tells me, *tourism is my passion.*

Sipping our mineral water, while facing the street, we discuss beauty and style and she tells me that her Aunt Odile is her true role model. *My mother's life was broken the day my father left her, when I was a baby,* Frédérique says, *so I had to find a model of how a woman should be—someone who takes care of herself.* And then, Frédérique describes her Aunt Odile. She is sixty-seven and very active. She loves to bicycle, she hikes, and she's interested in music and the arts. Frédérique's aunt is divorced like her mother, and never remarried. And while the two sisters were raised the same way, Frédérique believes they are very different. While her mother never recovered from the demise of her marriage, Odile has thrived.

I take care of my skin because of her, Frédérique says, and then tells me how her aunt instructed her when she was a teenager, *you have to begin to take good care of your skin.* Frédérique began with Clinique's night cream and is still loyal to it today. She tells me this is partly because it's less expensive than many French creams. One of my favorite

questions to ask French women is what they like to buy
when they're in America. I'm especially interested in the
things they can get in the States that they can't buy in France,
because as Americans I think we often take our own trea-
sures for granted. And so, Frédérique tells me that she likes
to buy tops at Banana Republic. *They're very nice!* she says,
and then continues, *I learned style from my aunt—she
would choose a specific necklace with a specific top.*

And then I compliment Frédérique on her ensemble and
the lovely wooden beads. She says I must meet her aunt and
her aunt's friends in Rouen, which is just a few hours from
Paris. And so, we agree to meet in Rouen in a few days where
her aunt lives, so that I can meet her and interview her
myself.

I decide to take the train from Paris to Rouen and arrive
a few days before our meeting so that I have an opportunity to explore the city on my own. Rouen is an ancient
town, made famous because it's the place where Joan of Arc
was burned at the stake for leading the French army against
the English. In the center of the oldest part of the town,
there's a very modern church that has been constructed in
her honor. At nineteen years old the peasant girl *Jeanne
d'Arc*, had a vision from God. This was during the time of
the One Hundred Years' War. And so while the British be-
lieved *Jeanne d'Arc* was a traitor and insane to boot, the
French declared her a saint.

In the center of the city is a cobblestoned square surrounded by lots of restaurants and tourist shops. I'm staying
in a modest hotel nearby, so for my first evening I have dinner in the square and I end up sharing a pizza with a lovely
couple from Australia. I tell them my husband is in Cairns,

researching coral, and they tell me this is a wonderful town not far from where they live.

The next night, I venture a little farther and find an authentic French restaurant filled with locals. Although, not at first. I arrive at eight o'clock and the place is completely empty. At first, I think—oh, this isn't a very good restaurant. No one is here. The waiter gives me a questioning look and places me at a little table by the door. It's not a great spot in terms of ambience, but as it turns out, it's perfect for people watching and taking my time sipping my *kir royale apperitif*. In fact, by eight thirty the place is full. It's as if everyone received an invitation saying, *Dinner at nine. Dress code: informal elegance. Be sure to bring a date.* Or several dates, because actually, there are lots of groups of two or three couples. I don't see any table with just women; however, I do see one table where two men are having dinner together. I am waiting for my main course—I've ordered the lamb stew, and I wait and wait.

I feel a little bit ignored and I am beginning to take it personally, until I realize that everyone seems to be served their starters at around the same time at nine o'clock. By nine forty-five, we all have our main course and the place gets very loud. Everyone seems to be competing to be heard; they raise their voices and the wine-infused laughter adds a kind of theatrical crescendo to the night. And I feel as if I have played my small part in this little culinary extravaganza. We are all offered a cheese course—I decline—and then dessert—apple tatin—I accept. And finally coffee. Now, the restaurant grows calm and I even sense a post-dinner-*triste* (sadness) in the place. One by one, the tables empty and the ladies and men in their elegant outfits leave the restaurant, some actually kissing the restaurant's owner on each cheek and shaking his hand as if he were the director of this fabulous show and deserves to be congratulated on creating such a marvelous event.

And I am tempted to thank him, too, because by the time I get up from my table at midnight, I feel as if I am about to leave a very good party and I ought to thank the host for inviting me into his home to enjoy his wonderful food and entertainment.

The next day, Frédérique, along with her Aunt Odile—a very pretty woman who looks more like forty-seven than sixty-seven, picks me up in her car and whisks me away to the outskirts of Rouen.

Frédérique has given me an amazing gift. She has organized a little party at the home of Aline, her Aunt Odile's friend. Oh, and what a home it is—surrounded by hills and fruit trees and a lovely garden. The house itself is quite old, from the sixteenth century. As we get out of the car, we are greeted by Aline, her husband, Didier, and Aline's good friend, Françoise. After a few pleasantries, we enter Aline's living room, which is so charming, filled with antiques and such a sense of history. There are colorful tiled floors and a couple of Louis XIV chairs with embroidered seats. I take a seat on one of the chairs and I get out my little notebook. Frédérique has prepared them by saying that I am an American author and I am here to find out how women of a certain age in France stay so stylish and beautiful. Oh, and these women are beautiful, not because they look young, but because they look like they are *bien dans leur peau*. Happy in their own bodies. Didier, a handsome, white-haired gentleman with a wonderful smile, gives his wife, Aline, a little pinch on the cheek and then disappears into another room. For a moment, I think, she's blushing. And then I think, but really could she be blushing? She is in her sixties with pure white hair and a sweet face and I see that yes, she is, indeed, blushing.

Aline is slender and wears a matching jacket and straight skirt in a pale white, pink and gray flower design. This may sound busy, but the colors are so muted that all you notice is how simple and fresh it looks on her and how the white goes with her hair. She wears hardly any makeup—actually none that I can see, but she does wear a gold chain necklace and matching button earrings. We settle into our little circle of chairs, with Aline and Frédérique across from me and Aline's good friend Francoise to my right and Aunt Odile to my left.

Frédérique tells the women that I was Meg Ryan's assistant and apparently the French love Meg Ryan!

This is what the three French *femmes d'un certain âge* tell me. Aline, Odile, and Françoise laugh and begin talking quickly; it's hard to keep up with them. I do understand that these French ladies feel that Meg Ryan is very adorable, very natural, and very funny.

And then, I jump right in and ask what's their secret to *ooh la la*. They all look at me, completely confused. *What is this ooh la la?* Okay, perhaps this is really just an American expression for French women. I don't think French women actually look at one another and say, *attention, girlfriend! You've got a lot of ooh la la going on today!* And so, I reframe the question and ask where they learned their sense of style. I get a different answer from each of the women. Aline says her mother taught her about style. Françoise says she learned style from looking at other women, and Frédérique's aunt Odile says that when she started to work and earn money, she became aware of the power of clothes. She tells me the story of how she bought a beautiful blouse with her very first paycheck. I listen as Odile describes this blouse, and as I watch her grow animated and passionate, I think—ah, this is the artsy woman in this little group of friends. She's the one with the braids and an amazing embroidered jacket that is so unusual. She tells us about her first purchase as if she bought it yesterday.

This blouse, she says, *it was very expensive. It was green with long sleeves, and small pleats. It had buttons in the back and when I wore it to work, people noticed it and I got so many compliments!*

Aline nods her head and agrees that what you choose to wear is very important. She tells me that she was a teacher for many years and *that if you want to tell children how to be, you must set a good example.* Odile adds, *the older you get, the more you have to take care of the package.*

Ah, "the package," and I imagine these women as three pretty party presents, wrapped up in bows. And then, Françoise tells me that when she first visited the United States, she wore her shoes with heels and she felt the men looking at her. They gave me the *regardez*, she says with a meaningful look. And this inspired her to dress well. And she still does. Today, she wears a crisp white skirt with a matching jacket, but the jacket is unbuttoned and so we can see that she is wearing a salmon and white-striped top. A new take on the French sailor shirt! Françoise reminds me of my cousin Beatrice, who is not a Vaillancourt like my French grandmother, but descended from the Couture side of the family. This makes me like her immediately.

The ladies get into a discussion on wearing skirts and dresses and heels and why it's important once you've retired to still get dressed up, go out, and be a part of the community. *And to keep your femininity!* Françoise says. *I wear skirts for my husband. He likes that.*

And then Aline adds, *I wear skirts, too, for my husband;* she whispers this because Didier is in the next room. And then she goes on to tell me how she was divorced in 1980 and was on her own for twelve years and then married Didier. *When I met Didier,* she explains, *I realized I could value my body. If nobody is telling you, sometimes you won't make an effort.* Ah, the power of love, I muse.

For their beauty regime, they *take the waters* a few times a year (meaning they go to one of the spas). And while Françoise and Odile go to the ones in Normandy, Aline says she prefers the ones in Spain and Germany. Oh, and they also take gymnastics classes. These are something like our old-fashioned aerobics classes, but a little less strenuous. It's more like a stretch and ballet class.

Odile says she likes to bicycle, and then she tells us how she has a hairdresser who comes to her house once a week. *I pay a reasonable price and she shampoos, dries, and braids my hair. Sometimes she does French braids and sometimes she does African braids.* And these braids look wonderful on her. I love the fact that these three women are so different in their styles, and yet such close friends. And once again, I am reminded of my dinner the night before and how this dinner was an event that we all shared. There was such a sense of community, and I suddenly see the idea of wearing a pretty green blouse, or getting your hair braided, as something you do to connect yourself to the larger world. We are all in this together, after all.

Next, I ask each woman to imagine that they have been working in the garden all morning and they are quite a mess, but they receive a call that someone is about to visit. They have five minutes to get ready. *What would you do?* I ask. *What's most important?*

All three women immediately answer, *lipstick!* Then they tell me that the second most important thing to do is to fix your hair, and the third most important thing would be to put on a bit of jewelry and if there's time, quickly change your clothes.

Next, I ask about perfume. Aline loves Miss Dior. She has been wearing it for forty years. She tells me, *I tried to change it once, but it didn't work. C'est impossible.* (It's impossible.) Odile, Frédérique's artistic aunt, says she changes her perfume every few years. Right now, she's wearing Yves St. Laurent's Cinema. *Because I love the cinema and also it's very pleasant and discreet.*

Francoise tells us that she doesn't wear perfume at home because her husband doesn't care for it, but she wears something light when she goes out. All through this, I can't help thinking how nice these ladies are to invite me over and to allow me to ask these seemingly shallow questions, but truthfully, I cannot ask them what I really want to ask them, which is to look at me and help me.

Make me French! I want to say. *I am a French American who has lost her way. My ancestors came to the New World in the 1600s and somehow the family lost the secrets des femmes. Please help me! Adopt me! Take me into the French fold—just give me a year with you and I'll do all your cooking and cleaning! I'll be your au pair! Just help me find my way back home.*

Of course, I say none of this, but instead, I pose this question—what would they do if an American girl came to them for beauty advice. I describe a worst-case scenario—an American girl who has messy hair and bad posture and dresses badly and is basically completely clueless about style and beauty. Odile looks at me or looks right through me and declares, *oui, but this girl—she must want to change.* I say, *okay, yes, she wants to change,* and I wonder if I'm talking about myself on some level, even though I do not have messy hair or clothes and I dress well enough and have decent posture. But I suppose I am really asking these women to have a conversation between the *femmes* and my earlier, younger self.

Françoise, the one who looks like my cousin Beatrice says, *I would bring her in front of the mirror to show her what she can change and how she can move her body.* Aline says she would teach her to be clean. *Even if she is wearing jeans and a T-shirt, she should be clean, with clean hair and clean shoes.*

I find myself a little frustrated because basically, their advice is quite simple and something any American mother would say to her daughter—sit up straight, wear clean clothes, take a look at yourself in the mirror. But, this mirror business reminds me very much of my French friend Tania's home. I often stay with her and I've noticed how she has placed a very large mirror on the wall at the end of her dining room table, so that when she sits at the head of the table, which she generally does, she faces herself in the mirror as she eats her dinner. It sounds simple, but perhaps this idea of mirrors is quite powerful. And I do think that we ought to put more mirrors across America. Everywhere—in our own homes, yes, but also in more stores and shops and in elevators and even at the Stop and Shop. Oh, and definitely at Target and Marshalls. Have you ever noticed how few mirrors they have? What's that about, anyway? Well, I have my theories.

But that's for another day, because the ladies and I are now on to diets. Who says French women don't diet? Aline tells us how she would like to lose ten kilos, and her doctor recommended she just have soup for dinner, and more fruits and vegetables. There's nothing new here, nothing exotic. And truthfully, to my American eyes Aline already looks quite slender. *My doctor said if I want to eat cheese, I should have it in the morning. And no sugar in the coffee.*

The ladies bustle around the kitchen preparing the meal. Each one, it seems, has contributed something to the feast. I am instructed to sit at the table and relax. And then, it's time for our dinner. Or lunch, but really dinner because their midday meal is the main one of the day, generally speaking.

And what a beautiful table they've prepared with pretty white dishes and gleaming silverware on a white tablecloth with candles and little crystal wineglasses. Didier, Aline's husband, tells me they've been in Aline's family for generations.

And then I notice that there are little butter knives poised on miniature silver animals. There's a dog, a rooster, a bird. It's so charming and I am so honored that they've gone all out for this luncheon! And then I am asked to sit down next to Didier, which I sense is the place of honor—almost as if they are saying, *You are the guest from America and so you get the treat of sitting next to the only man in the room!* Didier opens the bottle of white wine and pours a little in each glass, and we make a toast to *Les Femmes!* He tells me, *You see, Jamie, France is all about women!*

I look at him, wondering if he is just saying this to flatter the guests, but he continues. *It's true. France is the center of chic. We have Chanel, Dior. Fashion. Perfume. So, when a woman shops and buys clothes or perfume, it's supporting our economy. It's patriotic!*

Wow. Buying perfume is patriotic. I never thought of that before.

Aline sits down and looks around at the table. She seems pleased by how beautiful everything is, but then she realizes she has forgotten something. The salt! She quickly gets up from the table and then walks to the kitchen. Her back is turned to me and this is when I notice that her skirt's zipper in the back is unzipped. I can see her pale pink slip. Just a peek of something silky and fine. And at the same time that I notice this, Didier seems to have noticed this dishabille as well, because he quickly, wordlessly, gets up from the table and follows his wife. I cannot help watching as he stands behind her so that her unzipped skirt is no longer visible. And then, Didier gently places his hand on Aline's shoulder and whispers something in her ear, before he ushers her into the kitchen. I watch as the two of them discreetly disappear. It is a fine moment—a glimpse into the intimacy of a married couple. A couple that has been married for a long time. Somehow this unzipped moment is mesmerizing. It is a vulnerable moment, for sure, but it is also so ordinary and yet it's so poignant. But also, Didier's attentions make this scene so sexy and powerful. Honestly, if I were a writer of erotica, I would begin my story right here. An unzipped zipper. A husband's hand. A kitchen that is unseen by guests. And a sweet silk slip.

But, it's the fragility of the moment that truly makes it so sexy. Aline cannot see that her skirt is unzipped and her pink slip is showing. And I suspect that her husband's expert fingers at the back of her skirt must recall forgotten moments from many, many years ago, when her grandmother wore an old-fashioned corset and it was tied or untied by her grandfather while he stood behind her, pulling the lace through the eyelets and tying it so that it was just right.

And then, the moment is over. Aline and Didier return. And as Aline places the salt on the table, I see that her skirt is now properly zipped. Didier sits next to me and offers me some bread with pâté and some prunes made from their very own plum trees. And the meal begins as if nothing has happened. And I suppose nothing has happened, except in my own mind. Because for me, after all this searching and questioning, I have received an important clue to the secret to *ooh la la*.

We transfer the handicap and make it an asset!

If you recall, this is what Madame Josie Mermet told me in Paris. I think of it now because Aline's unzipped skirt has made me think of my mother. My mother was handicapped after we were in a terrible car accident. I was eight and she was thirty-eight, and while I was fine, my mother nearly lost her life. After many operations, the doctors were able to save her, but she was handicapped for the rest of her life. Her left leg was an inch shorter than her right leg and she always walked with a cane. She needed help with the most simple things like tying her shoes. I have a vivid memory of my father bending down and tying my mother's shoes for her, watching his fingers expertly tying her shoelaces into a double knot so they would be secure and not come undone. This may be something we take for granted, but when one has trouble with just walking, a secure shoelace can mean everything.

So how was her handicap an asset? Well, she took nothing for granted. Although walking was difficult, she liked to swim. And in her sixties, she took up horseback riding. Oh, and she never gave up tap-dancing—after all, she still had a very good right leg! All this is to say, her handicap became her asset. It made her plucky and wise and inventive and yes, full of *ooh la la.*

So here I am, at the dining room table, drinking red wine with a group of French people, and I am so happy. Somewhere in my mixed-up brain, Aline is my mother and Didier is my father, and I feel that ocean between us growing smaller and smaller moment by moment.

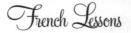

French Lessons

Take care of the package by paying attention to the little things in your life. Listen to the femmes d'un certain âge and sit up straight, comb your hair, put on a bit of lipstick, a fragrance, some clean clothes. This may sound terribly simple, but the truth is, when you take care of the details, you don't have to worry about the bigger picture. You don't need a major transformation, a face-lift, a wardrobe makeover, or a beauty intervention on a television show.

The day may come when you are swept up into unforeseen circumstances. Big or small. However, if you have taken care of yourself, a little every day, you will be able to ride the storms of fortune. And this is true, whether you have a serious accident or simply an unzipped zipper. This is because the habit of self-care, over a lifetime, prepares you for all the fortuities that life will present to you.

And perhaps, you'll even see this unexpected happenstance as a gift and a great opportunity to see your world anew.

And finally, feel the love! Be nice to your man and wear a skirt or a fine silk slip for him. It's a simple way to say I love you.

!!!

CHAPTER TWELVE

Le Mystère des Femmes

A wise woman never yields by appointment. It should always be an unforeseen happiness.

—STENDHAL

MADAME POUPIE CADOLLE is nothing like I expected.

And I suppose, I expected a lot. After all, she is the Queen of Lingerie! Her Great-great-grandmother, Madame Herminie Cadolle, created the first bra in 1889 and Madame Poupie Cadolle is the sixth generation of this family-run company, designing some of the most beautiful lingerie in the world. So, as it were, I am going to meet authentic *Lingerie Royalty*.

However, the arrangements take a few days to organize.

It is a Thursday afternoon in Paris and I make my way from Métro Opera to Boulevard de la Madeleine and cross the intersection to reach the most famous fashion street in all of Paris, rue de Cambon. It's here where you'll find the ghost of Madame Coco Chanel still walking the street and imperiously demanding that the visitor forget about Cadolle and notice her artfully decorated *atelier* and shop. After all,

Chanel is the one with the irrefutable legendary name, plus her windows are arranged in such a way that you simply can't ignore the fact that you are face to face with history. In the dazzling sunlight, it is almost too bright to see, and you must squint your eyes to focus on the larger than life (certainly taller than life) mannequins posing in their imperiously beautiful dresses, all with the same sleek black hair, looking down on you—in fact, staring down at you, as if reprimanding you for being short and American. And you turn and out of the corner of your eye, there's Coco herself, wearing her trademark boxy jacket and little hat, puffing on a cigarette and whispering something about you also being a bit on the bosomy side.

Yes, I am just imagining this last part.

And I do have a mission to find out the secret to the power of lingerie. And so, without too much effort, I am able to pull myself away from the specter of Chanel, and there— just across the street on the cooler, shaded side of rue Cambon, I find refuge from the blazing September sun in front of Cadolle. The windows are filled with sweet candy-colored silk delicacies, nestled between black lace brassieres, all promising a night of unbridled passion. I stand there, with exactly the same feeling I have when standing in front of a display of colorful macarons or raspberry-filled tarts that glisten ruby red. I am hungry for these little brassieres and matching panties. I want to take them home by the armful and fill my closets with these yummy treats. I don't even care whether they'll fit me or not!

And then I look over my shoulder and see Madame Chanel across the street, puffing on her cigarette and tsk-tsking at my big American appetite and my love for all things sweet.

Nonetheless, I brace myself. I swing open the door and

enter Cadolle. Ah, and I am not disappointed. The interior is a dark chocolate, filled with wooden cupboards half opened, revealing creamy pink and blue silk chemises edged in black lace, hanging delicately from silk, padded hangers with little bows at their hooks.

Before I let myself get too enraptured, I tell the young saleslady that I am an American author and ask whether it is possible for me to meet with Madame Cadolle. She tells me that I will need to make an appointment *avec Madame*. Then the girl takes out a large leather appointment book, flips a page, and looks for a date.

And in the meantime, I look around at all the silk robes and tiny lace-fringed panties. The air is so fragrant with perfume, you might think you've entered a very beautiful, very wealthy woman's boudoir. While I'm waiting, a young salesman comes up to me and asks me where I'm from. I find myself whispering, almost as if we are in a church and must be very quiet, so as not to disturb the precious silk chemises. I softly say I am from Cape Cod. Before he can ask me where that is, the saleslady returns and hands me a shiny black card with the name CADOLLE embossed in gold script lettering. She tells me that Madame will see me on Tuesday. I say *merci* again and *au revoir* and then tiptoe out of the store and into the brilliant sunshine.

Oh, and Madame Chanel is now nowhere to be seen.

I should explain that there are two different ways that one can buy lingerie at Cadolle. The store that I just visited is actually the ready-to-wear shop. And this is where you can pick out a bra or panties or a chemise or robe or slip or corset or garter belt. You can try it on and purchase it. This will not be cheap, but it will be a whole lot less expensive than the handmade lingerie in which you are measured by Madame Cadolle herself and your lingerie is made specifically for you in her *atelier* (her workshop/office) around the corner at the *haute couture* shop on rue Saint-Honoré.

This is what my friend Luanna did and how I originally found out about Cadolle. I met Luanna at the French Library in Boston and she told me how she first met Madame Cadolle in 2001. This was during the days when the boutique was still on the second floor of the rue Cambon address and there was a tiny elevator (slightly rickety, by all accounts) that could carry only one person at a time. Over the years, Luanna bought four handcrafted brassieres from Madame Cadolle—the most recent is made of Chantilly lace, which she happened to be wearing the evening I met her at the library. Luanna told me how she took her mother with her for her seventy-fifth birthday, which I do believe is a lovely birthday gift for one's mother. I know if my mother were alive, she would leap at the chance to visit Cadolle in Paris.

Personally, I've always adored good lingerie. I suspect this has something to do with my fascination with showgirls, the Folies Bergères, and the Moulin Rouge and all things frilly and feminine. I remember reading French fashion magazines as a twelve-year-old girl when I babysat for a woman doctor. She was a divorcee, and very sophisticated and exciting. Every Saturday night, as soon as her two boys were asleep, I would devour her copies of *French Vogue*, and later when I was home, I would pretend I was one of the models and drape myself in lace curtains from our linen closet that I had refashioned into a thrilling peignoir set and a bridal veil. It was a cross between a wedding gown and a honeymoon ensemble. Once my mother caught me posing in front of the full-length mirror in the hall and looked at me a bit alarmed and said, *what are you doing with the curtains!?*

I think I said something like, *pretending to be a fairy princess*, because that seemed like the most acceptable response. But in truth, I was pretending to be a French fashion model! And so this is how I began my illustrious (though largely unknown) career in lingerie.

On the appointed Tuesday, I walk around the corner from rue Cambon to rue Saint-Honore and then through a cobblestoned courtyard, tucked in away from the street, where I come upon a dark burgundy red awning with the name CADOLLE spelled out in gold.

Madame Cadolle's assistant asks me to wait in the reception area, and then within a few minutes I am escorted into a large room awash in pretty pinks and whites. Off to one side, there's a dressmaker's form draped in a half-made white corset with white lace ribbons floating across her bodice. Behind the form, I notice a velvet-draped dressing room, and right by it, a large three-way mirror. And this is by a very ornate antique sofa.

And then Madame Cadolle arrives, bustling into the room. She greets me warmly, taking my hand in hers. She is nothing like I imagined! She is downright cute and she has the sweetest smile. She is very blond and curvy and soft. She wears a simple black dress and a little printed black and white jacket— and plain flat shoes. No strappy stilettos, but something very practical. She tells me how happy she is to meet me and asks me to sit down. I thank Madame Cadolle and she says *please, call me Poupie.* And even this name, which sounds a little like *puppy* to my ears, adds to the feeling that I have just met a long-lost friend—the kind of friend you want to tell all your love problems to and then ask if she could possibly whip up a bra and a corset that will reframe your body into something luscious and perfect and sexy and make you feel brand new again, oh, and solve all your problems. And perhaps make you French, too.

But there's no time for these imaginings, because Madame is off running, telling me about black lace. She prefers black lace. And she has strong opinions. She doesn't like nude so much as black. Madame should certainly have a right to her opinions; after all, she makes over five hundred and fifty made-to-measure bras each year and fifty girdles. Yes, apparently French women do wear girdles. Plus, Madame Cadolle makes lots of traditional lace-up corsets. And her clients include movie stars and showgirls from the Crazy Horse.

The Crazy Horse, I repeat, and Madame gives me one of the French shrugs. *Why not?!* She looks at me from behind her very crowded antique desk and continues.

Here in France, we have no complex with beautiful lingerie.

And then she tsk-tsks at some long-ago slight from someone who apparently did have a complex when it came to beautiful lingerie. *It's a huge mystery over what's happened in the last fifteen years in America,* she tells me. I nod my head in sympathy, although I'm not exactly sure what she means. *The women in America want seamless, smooth bras with no lines. So you shouldn't even guess they have on a beautiful bra.*

Madame looks at me with great dismay. I nod my head in agreement, feeling a little bad that my compatriots have not stepped up to the plate when it comes to high-end lingerie.

She leans forward and continues. *You see, for some*

women—the sin is to show you have any beautiful lin-
gerie on. These women are closing the door to not just sexy,
but to all the pretty details.

I am frantically writing all this down in my little notebook.
Madame picks up and fingers a sheer white, lace-edged
brassiere on her desk. *You see,* she says, *French girls wear*
a pretty bra. It's not to be sexy. It's to be pretty, for them-
selves.

I am writing this down, but also I'm thinking she is really
onto something here, because it does seem that in America,
there is a great divide when it comes to lingerie. It is either
very utilitarian—cotton panties in three packs bought at the
supermarket at a discount, or some sexed-up itsy-bitsy biki-
nis in wild patterns along with big padded bras and laced-
up bustiers that are really just for show, because they actually
do nothing to enhance or smooth out a normal woman's
body. Although, admittedly they do look great on a twenty-
two-year-old, six-foot-blond model, with absolutely no body
fat—oh, and wings, because she's such an angel. An angel to
a fella in her bed, that is.

So, ultimately it seems to me that when we are wearing
undergarments for ourselves, our choice is to be utilitarian,
but without beauty. And when we are wearing undergarments
for our man, we can have beauty, but these beautiful little
nothings are kind of useless in terms of our own everyday
life. So, there's this strange disconnect. Madonna or Harlot?
You have to make a choice, I guess.

Oh, but yes, we do have contouring devices and thank heaven
for Spanx, but why can't they be prettier? Honestly, do we
really want to be seen in *dishabille* wearing only our Spanx?

But, here in France—here at Cadolle—you can have your
cake and eat it, too!

You can get a corset that is not only beautiful, lacy, romantic, and very, very pretty, but something that really does help a woman define her shape and feel gorgeous, smooth, and, dare I say, slim! Imagine this: Spanx meets Victoria's Secret made in sizes and styles for grown-up ladies with all the complications that happen to a body past the age of twenty-five. And you'll find these lovely underthings, not just at the high-end haute couture shops, but even at the French department stores, as well as the little lingerie shops in the tiny villages where a sweet older lady will measure and assist you.

Madame tells me that in France it's all about aesthetics, and this has been the case since the Renaissance. *You see, she says, our eye is built for beauty.*

So what happened in America? I ask. *Why don't we seem to appreciate good lingerie, just for ourselves the way the French do?*

And she tells me that she believes that when the Europeans immigrated to the New World—a rugged, unsettled place—they had to forget their European roots, just to survive.

For a moment, I imagine the first settlers in Plymouth and how the niceties of lingerie and perfume must have seemed so frivolous in the face of the frigid winters and starvation. I think of my French ancestors in Canada and how very, very cold that first winter must have been. How many people died on just the voyage over? Lots, I'm sure. And how many were lost during the first years in the New World? I'm sure there were many. And so, I understand something about my own country's distrust for female fineries. In this context, things like lace panties and matching bras seem indulgent and perhaps even dangerous.

And now, Madame becomes sad. She cannot understand our American penchant for smooth-smooth-smooth. Bras without seams, panties with no visible lines. *I don't understand this,* she says. *We have seams, lace, embroidery! You can guess there's something pretty underneath.* She gives me a bewildered look. *The American woman says, "I don't want someone guessing what's underneath!"*

And I think, of course the American woman doesn't want anyone to guess what's underneath. Of course it's Victoria's or Suzie's or Madeline's secret—because wearing good lingerie is actually kind of naughty in a country that was founded, not too long ago in relative terms, by a bunch of really tough guys (and gals), wearing furry pelts and coonskin hats. But, somehow I can't explain this to her.

Madame continues.

Even in New York, they think lace is a sin. Women in the United States have a uniform for running. And the uniform for sleeping with a man. But that uniform is for the man, not for them. It's for a special occasion. There's no romance there, because they are "ready." This way of wearing lingerie is too organized.

And then, we are talking about the politics of men and women. Madame Cadolle feels we have gone too far in America. And she tells me that we have built a "wall" between men and women. Her cheeks flush pink as she tells me, *in the elevator, a man smiles and suddenly there's a lawsuit. Men are frightened of women. Women have the power, the money, and men are not even allowed to smile, compliment, or touch.*

I tell her that this is not completely true and that it's a complete exaggeration, but never mind, because somehow all the French people I talk to—especially the French men— seem to think that all we do in America is file sexual harassment lawsuits against every single unwitting, Don Juan wannabe. Oh, and on top of this, the French seem to have this idea that the sexual harassment lawsuit always begins in an elevator when a man looks at a woman and says something as innocent as *your hair looks nice today.* As a result, French men are petrified of riding in American elevators. So, if you ever find yourself in an elevator in America with a French man, don't be hurt if he just stares at the wall in front of him and doesn't look at you, or talk to you.

Next, Madame tells me that women in the United States will sit at a bar and it's perfectly fine for a strange man to start talking to her, and then she shakes her head and says, *but if he works with her, he can't!* She shrugs her shoulders and continues. *A French woman would never sit alone in a bar.*

I must admit, she's onto something. So, it's okay for a stranger to flatter us, but it's not okay for someone we actually know to flatter us. That is kind of weird, in a way, yes?

And then, she tells me how French husbands come in with their wives for the custom-made lingerie, and she describes how for the couples it's such a special occasion. The woman tries on her lace corset in the dressing room and then he sits in the antique chair—and the man takes a great interest in the lingerie.

For the man, it is important that he choose his wife's lingerie. Even if it's far from her style, the fact that she's wearing something he chose for her makes him think of her.

And then Madame tells me that American men never accompany their wives or girlfriends for the fittings, and that the women not only come in by themselves, but also pay for everything themselves.

A couple of weeks ago, I had an American couple here,

but the American man doesn't pay any attention. He's reading The New York Times.

I tsk-tsk at this, and not just to empathize with Madame, but because it does seem like a shame to me, and a lost opportunity for a husband and a wife to bond. And yet, I don't know if I'd want my husband watching me get fitted for some sexy (yet, completely practical) lingerie. I am an American woman, after all. But, as Madame describes the process of being fitted, the beautiful fabrics, the perfect measurements, and choosing the perfect colors for the individual woman (she does seem to favor black lace), I must admit I am drawn in. I want to be that woman—the woman who is admired by her husband in a pair of those specially made undies. And then, Madame says the one thing that really seals the deal for me. She describes how she has a few clients—couples in their sixties and seventies—who have been coming to her for years. *That old?* I want to say, but I don't. Still, she can see by my expression that I am impressed by this.

Of course, why not? she says. *French women never stop wanting to be beautiful.* And then, she looks deep into my eyes and says, *we are here to make all women feel beautiful.*

And I know in this moment we are talking about everything—age and size and insecurities and handicaps, and all those little things that conspire to make a woman feel shy or not beautiful or not deserving of a six-hundred-dollar corset.

Okay, yes. It's six hundred dollars. (The panties cost eighty dollars each.) But, imagine this. It's a couture corset that is designed and sewn and tailored and re-tailored, using fabric and colors and details that are specifically created just for you. It's a one-of-a-kind piece of original art that you wear on your body. And you keep it forever, because yes, it's that well made.

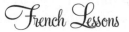

Back in 2007, when my good friend Jessica Lee and I traveled all over France together conducting interviews, we asked French women (and lots of men) what is your secret to confidence? How do you find love? How is it that you've earned this reputation for beauty and intrigue? And most importantly what's the secret to ooh la la?

The first answer we always got—whether the group consisted of twenty-five women or two women or one individual woman—was, in one word, lingerie.

Yes, lingerie!

And then they would tell us—the bra and panties must always match.

Jessica and I found this so simple it was absurd and we would laugh and shake our heads. Why must they always match? Who's to know? I would ask, and the French women would shake their heads and look at us with great seriousness and say—why, you would know! Simple!

Now, it's been quite a few years since these first interviews and I've come to realize that the secret to ooh la la *is not really so simple. Yes, lingerie is a part of it, but it goes much deeper. The French woman's confidence, her* ooh la la, *comes from the place within her psyche that would make her want to buy good lingerie. Ooh la la is not so much lingerie or perfume or fashion. These are the outward expressions of something that goes much deeper. The question to ask then is not what is* ooh la la, *but where does* ooh la la *come from? And the answer is—lots of places. It comes from her life experience, her childhood, her family, her education, her attitudes, her travels, her friends, her triumphs, her failures. It comes from the books she reads, the movies she sees, the days she walks in the park. It comes from her daydreams and her dinner parties. It comes from life and loss and love.*

And yes, it comes from wearing fine lingerie next to her skin every day. Oh, and you don't have to buy the most expensive underwear in the world, but consider wearing something pretty every day. You'll see—you'll feel the difference. And the world will reflect this back to you in a million wonderful ways.

!!!

CHAPTER THIRTEEN

My Perfect Moment

And now here is my secret, a very simple secret: It is only
with the heart that one can see rightly; what is essential
is invisible to the eye.

—FROM *Le Petit Prince*

WHEN JESSICA LEE first learned that I'd become close to her
French friend, Tania, she was really surprised. *You and Tania?!
But you're so different! And you're going on a road trip
together? Really?!*

Jessica Lee is the one who first introduced me to Tania.
Jessica was working for a French company in Connecticut,
and Tania spent a year there before returning to France. I
met Tania in 2007 and yes, we are very different, but I think
that's why we get along so well. She's a businesswoman—
organized, efficient, and very opinionated in that very French
sort of way. I am none of these things. However, I love that
she is! Truly, she's the quintessential French girl. And I have
so much to learn from her. The thing is, I am almost Tania's
mother's age. Actually, I'm also almost Jessica Lee's mother's

age. If I were a teenage bride, they could be my daughters. I think this makes a difference when I meet up with the French girls. We seem to have a kind of mother-daughter relationship that I find very comfortable.

Anyway, Tania is a beautiful girl. Smart. Very chic, and also quite formidable. I think that's why I'm crazy about her, too. She makes me want to be a better person. I cannot be lazy around Tania.

On the day of our road trip, before we leave for Normandy, for lunch we make an endive salad with fresh walnuts that she brought back from her parents' home in the country. She makes her salad dressing using a big silver tablespoon and fills it about a third with olive oil and then a drop of mustard, which she mixes in and then fills up the rest with balsamic vinegar.

I ask her how she learned to do this, and she looks at me as if everyone makes their salad dressing this way. And then, sweetly (because I am just an American after all, which means I am just a child—although this is probably my imagination), she tells me that her mother taught her to make it this way. And in fact, the big silver spoon originally belonged to her grandmother, then her mother, and now it is hers. We sit down to our salads and baguette and little slices of *jambon* (ham), and then Tania pours just a little white wine into the tiny glasses she recently bought from the *vide grenier*—the town-wide annual tag sale that takes place in her local park. At first, I am a bit worried. We are going to drink wine and then we are going to drive all the way to Normandy? But, the wine in these glasses—it's about a thimbleful. And I understand. This wine is delicious, a little treat—like a tiny square of good dark chocolate and that's all. No second glasses, no big goblets that will send you into la la land. Just a little taste and you don't need any more than that.

After all—France awaits us!

And then, we fetch Tania's car—we gas it up—fifty euros to fill the tank—or about seventy-five dollars. And we're not talking about an SUV, but a little European sporty car. So, you see, this is a special occasion. It is not inexpensive and it's a little like the wine at lunch or the chocolate. It's precious, so we don't overdo.

And then we're in the countryside!

Ah, the green. I am so excited about going to Normandy, because I've never been there and because this is where my French ancestors are originally from. To be precise, they come from the little village in the northwestern part of France called Saint-Nicolas-d'Aliermont.

I am here because my ancestors, the Vaillancourts, are originally from this little village. But more than this, I am waiting for what the late actor/writer Spalding Gray describes in his monologue *Swimming to Cambodia* as his search for the Perfect Moment. My secret fantasy is that I will meet a Vaillancourt. A wise woman. She will invite me into her home and we will realize that we have so much in common and then perhaps she'll invite me to move in and I will get an education on *ooh la la* and then come home six months from now, completely transformed. Oh, and brimming with *ooh la la.*

And so when Tania turns into a road that directs us to the village of Saint-Nicolas-d'Aliermont, I get goose bumps. I really do. I am so happy to be in this place that has a connection to my past. Oh, and it's a sweet little village. We drive in and right there in the center stands the Cathedral Saint-Nicolas-d'Aliermont. It was built in the fifteenth century and is so beautiful. My cousin, Gloria Moreau (she's on the Couture side of the family and her husband is also French), did the genealogy and found out that our ancestors were married in this cathedral in the sixteen hundreds.

Tania pulls her car into the parking lot of Hotel du Commerce and we go to the little café/bar in the front to register and get our keys. This is the only hotel in the town of Saint-Nicolas-d'Aliermont, and Tania felt it was very important that I actually sleep in the town where my French ancestors are from. This hotel is more of a restaurant that happens to rent out a few rooms. Tania and I bring our bags up the stairs where we each have a little room with a single bed. The bathroom is down the hall. I get the feeling that we are the only ones staying in the hotel, and indeed when we come back downstairs to ask about the town, we get some very curious looks.

Oh, you're American! the manager exclaims. Apparently, he doesn't meet many Americans in this part of the world. I tell him that my grandmother was a Vaillancourt and that I'm here to see where my ancestors came from. He tells me that unfortunately there are no Vaillancourts in this town. I feel my Perfect Moment fading away. Tania and I walk across the street to the cathedral, but it's closed. It is Saturday afternoon after all. Still, it's disappointing. We walk about town a bit and I fantasize about moving here. There is a hairdresser, of course, and a *boulangerie* and *charcuterie*. There's an old clock factory that's empty and boarded up, and across the street is an abandoned chateau. It's quite beautiful, with huge windows and a brick wall all around it, overgrown with plants and tangled-up trees. It's something out of Dickens's Miss Havisham's house. I tell Tania that I am going to buy it, restore it, and move to Normandy. Of course, I'm just kidding, but the thought lingers in the air. Tania and I walk back, greeting stray cats walking in the middle of the road and looking at the pumpkins in the backyards, the flower gardens. It's a quiet town and very sweet.

When Tania and I return to the hotel, there is another man waiting at the front desk for me. *Are you the Vaillancourt?* he asks me. I say yes and he tells us that there's a rue de Vaillancourt just up the street. I am so excited, I can't quite contain myself. Tania and I get into her car and drive to the street. Yes, there it is. I get out of the car and she takes pictures of me standing beside the sign.

Tania says that the Vaillancourts must have been very important people to get a street named after them. Somehow, I don't think this is the case, but a part of me wants to believe it. I do know the Vaillancourts came from Normandy to Quebec in the 1600s on the Cartier expedition. And I do know that my grandmother used to say they lived in a place called Peche. I mention this to Tania and she explains that peche means fish and it's just a generic term for any town near a marina. And so, we drive over to Dieppe—a nearby town, southwest of Saint-Nicolas-d'Aliermont. We eat lots of cold snails, dipped in garlic mayonnaise—I know it sounds weird, but it's actually really good. They're called *bulots.* They're much bigger than escargot and very pretty. After this we have some *moules à la marinière* (mussels) and finally a salad and cheese course.

After dinner, Tania and I walk along the marina. The water is dark and swirling. It's getting cold outside now. I love the smell of the ocean, the salty smells. I try to imagine what it was like hundreds of years ago and what kind of people my ancestors were. They must have been hardy, that's for sure.

And the truth is, I feel very little connection. This idea that my ancestors might give me the secret key to *ooh la la* now seems a little ridiculous. And perhaps what I'm really after is something else, something I can't quite put my finger on.

I fall asleep that night with the sound of rain and wind, and the next morning I wake up early and I am downstairs at the café before Tania. The breakfast comes included with the room—a little baguette, butter, jam, orange juice, and *café au lait*. And since today is Sunday, I am excited to go into the cathedral and talk to the priest and ask about the history, thinking perhaps this is where my Perfect Moment lies.

After a while Tania joins me; we have breakfast and we walk across the street to the church. Oddly, the parking lot is filled with a farmer's market. And then, we see why. When we reach the door to the church, there's a sign saying that their usual mass will be held at a neighboring church, and the doors are locked. I am really upset. It seems this trip has been somewhat foolish. We go back to the hotel and I ask for a phone book. I look for Vaillancourts. I find none. And then, the local police officer comes into the hotel and tells us he has a key and he will let us in to the church!

Ah, and what a church it is. At first it's dark and so it takes a few moments for my eyes to adjust. And then I gasp. It's very beautiful, with very old stone and stained glass windows. There are all sorts of signs written in Latin and pictures of saints. There is something so primitive about the place—from the uneven stonework to the little wooden chairs with wicker backs lined up neatly in little rows. I breathe in the cool air. The oldest part, built in the fifteenth century, is where the baptisms and marriage ceremonies took place. I stand before the baptismal circle and breathe in, trying to feel the presence of the Vaillancourts. I wonder if they feel me there, an American woman who has returned after five hundred years to find out about their homeland, to learn, perhaps, something of their lives. I say a little prayer as a way of greeting them through the centuries. And my heart grows still.

And then, at this exact moment, the door to the cathedral opens and a blast of light enters the room. An elderly man walks slowly forward and shouts out, *I hear there's a Vaillancourt in the church!*

C'est moi! (That's me!) Although, until this moment, I have never thought of myself, really, as a Vaillancourt.

But that is me. Although, that's not exactly me. But, never mind. After all, I am a granddaughter of a Vaillancourt. Close enough! The man approaches Tania and me and introduces himself. This man is about my father's age with pink cheeks and big ears and twinkling blue eyes. Oh, and he's quite a dresser, too. I tell him I'm from America and Tania adds that I am here looking for ancestors. He is a little out of breath and seems very happy to see us. He kisses me on the cheeks and tells me that he was so excited to meet a Vaillancourt. We sit down and he explains that I am not the first Vaillancourt to visit the cathedral. A few years ago, another Vaillancourt, from Canada, was here. *She was right here in our village, just like you!* he tells me.

And then, this man proceeds to tell me the most amazing story. *During the German occupation, our clock factory was turned into a prisoner-of-war camp and this Canadian Vaillancourt was captured. But then one day, he escaped and we found him in my neighbor's apple orchard, eating all his apples. He was practically naked and starving. And so we took him in and hid him.*

I wonder if this is why there's a rue de Vaillancourt. Did

he come back after the war? Did he help the town? But this man doesn't seem to know the answer to these questions. He was just a boy during World War II. For me, the story brings me back to my own early childhood memory of sitting on the couch in my grandparents' living room and listening to my grandmother whisper to my mother about a Canadian cousin who was captured during World War II. I never quite understood much about this story, and perhaps I don't understand much more now, but I feel as if a piece of a puzzle has been put into place for me.

And then, this man kissed me on each cheek again, as if welcoming a long-lost cousin. And for that moment, I felt as if I, too, had been a prisoner and he found me in his garden, naked, eating the apples. And then, the good people of Saint-Nicolas-d'Aliermont have opened their doors to me and clothed me and fed me, because I am so hungry. I haven't eaten from these gardens in five hundred years, and I am starving for the taste of home.

So, I am French after all. But, I just don't feel very French. I've lost the thread; I've lost my way home. And I think something essential was lost when my ancestors crossed the oceans and arrived in the new land all those many years ago. There was no time to hold on to the past, the traditions, the helpful things that grandmothers told us. The recipes, the little secrets that women share. After all, there was a new country to settle.

I think I'm not alone in this feeling of disconnection with one's homeland. This longing for something that has been lost—whether it's France or Spain or Italy or England or Africa or India or Jamaica or Brazil. We need to reconnect, but how?

But how?

I think the first step might be talking to our elders. Our grandmothers and great-grandmothers, if possible. And of course, traveling back to our homeland is a way to form a kind of roadmap to beauty, to self-knowledge. And this is what I am doing in France. Because while it might not make sense to everyone, for me, when I see a lady in the market wearing a red wool cape and a pair of black rain boots, carrying a little net bag filled with fresh tomatoes and leeks, I know that I am collecting clues into my own past, and my own inner life.

And yes, this meeting in this church with this old man is definitely my Perfect Moment. As we leave the church, I say to Tania—*so now you can see, I really am French,* and she looks at me, a little distracted. She is now buying a bunch of fresh carrots from the farmer's market outside.

She says, *Because you're wearing a scarf?*

And I say, *no!* And then I find myself in tears. *Because of what the man in the church said. Because I'm a Vaillancourt!*

And Tania shrugs slightly before handing her euros over to the vegetable seller. *Oh, but you were always a Vaillancourt, n'est pas?*

I've thought about this moment ever since. When I told Tania I was really French, she went directly to the idea of wearing scarves. And I thought, well, that sounds awfully superficial. There's more to being French than wearing scarves! But as we drove through the countryside on our way to Rouen, I began to ask myself, suppose being French is really just about wearing scarves? And suppose being French isn't really about being French, but about being one's own true self? With all this searching for *ooh la la*—have I really been looking for the answer to the question *who am I?* And I wonder if answering this question is actually the ultimate beauty adventure a woman can participate in. In a way, my search for ancestors is connected to what Josie Mermet said about identity. And so, searching for one's ancestors is very much connected to searching for your own beauty and style roadmap.

French Lessons

Don't wait for your perfect moment. Rather, step forward bravely and search for your heart's desire. In the searching, you will find your perfect moment and you will find your ooh la la. *But be prepared for the distinct possibility that your* ooh la la *might not be what you imagined. In fact, you just might find that your* ooh la la *is better than anything you could have imagined.*

Talk to your family. Your parents, your grandparents. Your aunts and uncles. Their stories are the little clues to your own history and the continuing journey through life. After all, we are all part of this great continuum. And we are all connected. The more you know about where you've been, the better idea you'll have about where you want to go. So, ask questions, look at old photos. Listen to the family stories—the real ones as well as the fantastical, made-up, exaggerated stories that are more like tall tales. All these narratives are your gold and your link to your own true self.

!!!

CHAPTER FOURTEEN

Are You an Audrey or a Marilyn?

And the day came when the risk to remain tight in a bud
was greater than the risk it took to bloom.

—ANAÏS NIN

IT'S SATURDAY NIGHT in Paris and the girls have gone wild!

Actually, truth is, two American girls are being just a little
bit wild on the streets of Belleville. This is a working-class/
emigrant neighborhood in the north of Paris where Edith
Piaf once lived. It's also an artsy place with lots of galleries
and cafés. And every year in June, you can come here to the
canals to enjoy the famous *fête de la musique* (festival of
music).

But here it is October, and Paris is getting awfully chilly.
It's been raining on and off since I arrived here, and I'm
afraid I'm now catching a cold. Still, even with that scratchy
feeling in my throat, I sing along with Elizabeth as we walk

along the canal. And so, the night is over and we are having an Edith Piaf moment. We croon together:

Il me dit des mots d'amour, des mots de tous les jours!
(He speaks words of love to me, words all day long.)

And since we can't remember the rest of the lyrics, we just blast out *"La vie en rose"*! And for some unknown reason, this makes us howl with so much laughter we have to hold on to each other so we don't fall into the canal. Possibly, it's just the wine, but more than this, I think it's from the giddiness of being together in—of all places—Paris!

I met Elizabeth back in 1996 at the Virginia Center for the Creative Arts. We were both on writing fellowships. We became good friends after a night of dancing to country western music at the Holiday Inn with a bunch of other VCCA artists along with the local cowboys. And we've been good friends ever since. And then, to everyone's surprise, she up and married a Brit and moved to England! But the nice thing about that is when I'm in Paris, she's only a chunnel ride away. And so here we are, sharing a studio rental right by the Cemetery Pere Lachaise. This is where you'll find the writer Collette, along with Oscar Wilde, Marcel Proust, Sarah Bernhardt, and Chopin. Oh, and Jim Morrison of the *Doors*. At night, from the studio, if you open the window really wide and listen very carefully—you can hear Jim crooning ever so softly, *Come on baby, light my fire*. And then, Chopin tells Jim to quiet down because he's giving him a headache. And then, Collette suggests poor Jim come over and sit by her.

Okay, not really.

But Elizabeth and I like to imagine all this.

And now here we are, walking down rue Beaurepaire, deconstructing all things French, specifically, what just happened at the dinner party we attended earlier in the evening.

We have just come from Restaurant Astier, where we were hosted by Terrence Gellenter, the expat/raconteur/bon vivant and author of *Bagels to Brioches*. We arrived a tad bit late and Terrence insisted that the two of us sit at opposite ends of a very long banquet table, and so Elizabeth and I had absolutely no opportunity during the meal to look at one another cross-eyed or to make a cryptic comment in English. Still, any cryptic comments in English would probably be easily understood because there were plenty of English-speaking French people and about five or six America women and men visiting Paris.

Terrence—who's lived all over the world, although he now calls Paris home, is a big film buff and knows just about anything you'd like to know about Hollywood. Especially, old Hollywood. And so, at one point in the evening, he began entertaining us with this very funny story about meeting the famous director Billy Wilder. Billy directed Marilyn Monroe in *Some Like It Hot*, and Audrey Hepburn in *Sabrina*. Terrence said he asked Billy Wilder what it was like and apparently Billy Wilder replied that after directing Audrey Hepburn, he thought this gal *may single-handedly make bosoms a thing of the past!*

Now, I'm not usually like this. But I was a bit swept away by the *ooh la la* that night and I must confess, I'm a huge Marilyn Monroe fan, plus, if we have to discuss body types, I'm a Marilyn, not an Audrey, and so I sat up and cupped my ample bosoms and said in response to this idea that they'll become a thing of the past, *I beg your pardon!?* Only a few of the people around me could see my gesture of cradling my bosoms, but it still got a huge laugh. And I laughed, too, and turned red, because I honestly have no idea where this came from. I don't even think Marilyn would have said this.

It was really more of a Mae West kind of line. It was definitely the kind of line you say while wearing a big blue feather boa you bought in Paris (which was actually still sitting in the shopping bag back at the studio by the Pere Lachaise cemetery).

Still, I do believe that something shifted for me that evening. And after all these weeks of chasing *ooh la la*, it kind of jumped up from behind and grabbed me that night at Restaurant Astier. I had somehow crossed over.

So, after a lot of delicious food and wine and conversation, Elizabeth and I walked all the way from the restaurant back to Belleville. A very long walk indeed. And while it was quite late, the bars and cafés were still in full swing. We stopped at one little restaurant where the bartender waved us in and offered us free cous cous. The band was playing a kind of Middle Eastern music with such soul we had to stay. We took a table and drank a kir and listened to the band. Everyone was so excited that we were two Americans in Belleville and wanted to know exactly where we came from. I said Cape Cod, but nobody knew where that was, so I said Boston and people got excited. *Go Red Socks!* And all that. But when Elizabeth said she's from England, but she's American, well, this was just very confusing, and there was laughter and the band began to play another song, while a girl got up and danced a kind of modified belly dance.

Later, we walked down the boulevard, talking about the evening and laughing. *Can you believe what I did at the restaurant?* I asked, referring to my Mae West moment.

And this is when Elizabeth said to me, *hey, you're only middle-aged once, so you might as well have fun!*

My friend Elizabeth is so brilliant. I stop for a second and look at her. *Seriously*, I say. *You're right. Why do people al-*

*ways say, you're only young once? The truth is you're also
only middle-aged once!*

She smiles. *And, you might as well have fun!*

*But, Elizabeth, you've tapped into something really deep.
It's Zen. We're only middle-aged once.* And then we both
look at each and we're silent for a full three seconds before
we burst out laughing again.

Later that night, I laid in bed and closed my eyes and
thought about this illusive thing called *ooh la la.* I felt it in
the Restaurant Astier and again with Elizabeth in the bar with
the music. But I can't say it's something I planned. It just
happened.

Why did I feel so different in France, as if I had permission to be a little daring, to say something a little outrageous—at least, outrageous for me? Why did I feel this sense
of permission to come out of the metaphorical closet and
be myself? Why do French women always feel permission to
be completely themselves?

Lying there, I felt like a dozen blind men trying to describe an elephant. One part says, *ooh la la* comes from em-
bracing pleasure, another part of me says, no, it's the lingerie.
Another part of me says it's the style you see on the streets,
and another part of me says it's all the mentors they have
in their lives. And now, I think—it's the dinner parties. The
repartee. Oh, and music!

And I know, it's all of these things, but I also know that
there is some central philosophy that connects these parts
to make a whole. I just haven't found it yet. And honestly,
the French women themselves don't seem to know what the
secret ingredient is. They simply know that this is how they
live in the world. This is how they find their *joie de vivre,*

their *ooh la la*. But, because they've always lived with this thing, this secret ingredient, they can't seem to identify it for me or explain it. And so my search continues. But in the meantime, I must get some sleep. I must get over this cold.

In the morning, Elizabeth and I have a breakfast of a baguette bought from the *boulangerie* (bakery) downstairs, with butter and jam and wonderful coffee. Elizabeth and I discuss Charlotte Gainsbourg. This is because I have become obsessed with Charlotte Gainsbourg's nose.

This isn't because it's such a perfect little hardly-there nose, I tell Elizabeth. *No, Charlotte Gainsbourg has a nose that you notice. It's long and elegant.*

Elizabeth agrees and adds, *it's also just slightly too big for her face. In fact, it kind of calls attention to itself.* And this is when Elizabeth goes into her animated speaking voice— the one she uses when she plays ventriloquist for Frank, her cat. *Hello there, I am Charlotte's nose! How do you do?!*

Elizabeth, as Charlotte's nose, sounds exactly like her orange tabby cat named Frank, so I can't help imagining the two of them having a conversation, and so I join in also using the *Frank* voice—which is kind of a pulpy crime noir Sam Spade detective voice, circa 1929.

It's the imperfection that makes Charlotte's nose so appealing, so stunning. I can't take my eyes off her face!

Ah, says Elizabeth/Frank/Charlotte's nose, *it's true! I have a fabulous nose!*

Charlotte Gainsbourg is the daughter of Jane Birkin (the famous actress and singer for whom Hermès invented the Birkin bag) and Serge Gainsbourg—the iconic French singer, actor, and director. He had a tragic life, played out in the headlines of the day. Oh, and he had a nose, too. In fact, this seems to be where Charlotte got her nose. And I suspect this is partly why she has never felt the desire to "fix" it. Her nose is her legacy.

I am still thinking about it two days later, when I pack my suitcases to leave for Toulouse. It seems to me that we all have these facial and physical legacies. It might be a little bump on a nose, or for that matter, some green flecks in a pair of brown eyes, or an odd streak of silver in a twenty-something's auburn hair or the little mole on your left shoulder—all these are gifts from your mother, your father, your grandparents, and for all you know, your ancestors going back a thousand years. So when we reshape our faces and shave away the little imperfections, we are also cutting away some of the fine threads that connect us to our family, to our past. Yes, we have the ability to create something brand new. A new face, a new body. And yes, we have the ability to transform an aging face into something seemingly youthful, unmarked, unscarred by time, but at what cost? And I suppose I feel passionate about this idea of protecting our facial legacies, because I have just started discovering my own facial legacies. When I think about it, my grandmother was a bit bosomy and so was my mother. Who knows, perhaps that Vaillancourt who lived in Saint-Nicolas-d'Aliermont five hundred years ago was also a bit on the bosomy side. And this makes me think that my *ooh la la* isn't something that I invented today, but it's part of a lineage that goes way, way back, just like Charlotte's nose.

And now, here I am with my suitcase at the bottom of the circular wooden staircase. I have said my good-byes to Elizabeth and I turn around one last time to look back and say a silent good-bye to Belleville. And that's when I see it—I don't know how I managed to miss it all this time, but there's a little sign at the bottom step that reads, *Essuyez vos pieds*

S.V.P. In this moment, I assume this means *Watch your step, please*. However, later I will realize the sign said *Wipe your feet, please*. In that moment, something registers in my brain. Perhaps something a little prescient, because I take that message in. I tell myself I should watch my step. I must be careful going up and down these crazy circular French staircases. And so, for the rest of this trip, I am very careful when it comes to climbing up or down staircases. I watch my step.

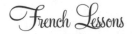

French Lessons

 Consider the power of the dinner party to find your ooh la la. *In the context of a group—whether you're hosting the party yourself, or meeting in a restaurant, it's an opportunity to try out your truest self. Dare to be a little theatrical or political or intellectual. Don't worry, nobody will let you go too far. But think of this as a way to get in touch with your essential self in the safety of friends and family.*

 Ask yourself, what is my facial or physical legacy? Have you, up to this point, thought of it as a flaw? Is it something that your mother or grandmother or aunt also has? Then, celebrate it. Find a way to turn that so-called flaw on its head and make it your fabulous trademark. Embrace and enjoy the things that make you different.

 And finally, bring music into your life. It has a wonderful way of shifting the molecules in your brain and making you see the world brand new.

!!!

CHAPTER FIFTEEN

Great Expectations

French women know they do not have control over the future.

—MICHELINE TANGUY

FROM PARIS, I take the train at Gare du Montparnesse to the south, through Bordeaux and on to Toulouse that evening. My French friend Beatrice—she's the one who gave me the strawberries and basil recipe for my first book—picks me up at the train station, and we catch up. I adore Beatrice! She has such a wonderful romance with her partner, Jean Pierre. He's in the French military and most recently went to Haiti to help the earthquake victims. He's such a calm and caring man. He's the one who will insist on holding your purse for you when you're walking through the rougher parts of town.

And yet, while Beatrice is very busy with her teenage son, and her handsome Jean Pierre, who, I've just learned, has had some medical issues, she still makes time for me. I sleep in a guest room that's downstairs. In the morning, I walk up the spiral metal staircase and greet Beatrice in the kitchen.

She's a very motherly kind of French woman. She wears little wire rim eyeglasses and she's fiercely intellectual. She has a Ph.D. from Yale University (yes, that Yale) and she speaks perfect English. This morning, she's wearing a long, flower-patterned linen nightie from Liberty of London (her favorite designer), but she's already on the phone, working.

Beatrice has a very high-stress job, although I am not exactly sure what she does. All I know is that there are piles of papers and folders and that she wears little earphones when she's talking on the phone and she's very intense. Still, she manages to fetch me a cup of fresh café from the kitchen. She places a baguette, some butter, and a jar of apricot jam from her mother's home in the country. And so my day begins.

My flight is scheduled to leave early Monday morning, but I have today to shop and then Sunday to pack and relax. When I walk down the spiral staircase in Beatrice's home, I am careful to hold on to the banister, but by the time I walk out her door and onto the cobblestone street, I have forgotten about being careful and so I blithely walk down the street and over to the main boulevard.

I love Toulouse. The south of France is so different from Paris. And it's really different from the north. As I'm walking down the rue Merly, past the cathedral at Place Saint-Sernin, I can't help noticing how women here wear more color and seem a little more relaxed than up north. Toulouse is known as "The Rose City" because all the buildings have a pink tone to them. And the light is so special. It's right on the banks of the Garronne River and not that far from Spain, so I think there's that influence. Plus there's all that sunshine and since Toulouse is a university town, it's fun to watch the students from the viewpoint of a café table at La Place du Capital, which is where I'm going now, because they have a wonderful outdoor market on Saturday mornings.

I spend the day going to the little tourist shops, buying souvenirs for my family and friends back home—violet liqueur, violet candy, and violet potpourri. Toulouse is famous for its violets, and besides I love to make violet kirs when I get home— that's white wine with a splash of violet liquor. It's sweet, but also perfumey. And besides, you just can't find this anywhere but in the south. I run about the city, taking lots of photos. I buy two Armand Thierry dresses. Thierry is a French designer and her things are not very expensive and always look nice on me. And then, I get my hair shampooed and "brushed out." But this time, I tell the hairdresser to leave in my natural curls. Finally, I buy a gift of really fine chocolates for Beatrice and Jean Pierre.

I am exhausted, but I am pleased at all I've accomplished and I'm looking forward to a nice dinner out.

As I walk back down Rue Lafayette toward Beatrice's home, I notice that the pavement is still a bit slick. Somehow I manage to get a little confused—the streets are so winding and narrow, and for a few minutes, I find myself walking in the wrong direction. I am now on Boulevard de Strasbourg, but nothing looks familiar. I feel a panic rising in my chest. A hot flash runs through me, up my arms, my throat, my neck, to my scalp.

I'm worried about being late for dinner. I do not have a cell phone, and even if I did have an international cell phone (which I don't, but should have), I have neglected to carry Beatrice's telephone number or even her address with me. It's been a long stay in France and I am going home on Monday, and so I think perhaps one part of me has already left the country and I am beginning to unravel a bit, just a bit.

Please, just get me through until the day after tomorrow, I think, and then I'll be meeting my husband at the Boston Logan Airport where we will then go to the Logan Airport Hilton. I will take a long luxurious bath. We will order room service. I will give him my gifts of Toulouse violet liqueur and packaged foie gras and I will show him what I bought for myself—the red boots, the perfume, the blue feather boa.

But right now, I'm lost! And it's beginning to get dark in Toulouse and the streets are wet. And it might rain again. I must get back to Beatrice's house. And so, I try to be rational. Since I do not recognize any of the shops on Boulevard de Strasbourg, perhaps this is because I am walking in the wrong direction. So even if this means I may be losing valuable time, I turn around and go in the opposite direction. And then, *voila!* I am back to where I began earlier in the day and everything looks familiar and I know exactly where I need to go.

And now, the three of us—me, Beatrice, and Jean Pierre—are going out for an evening on the town. It's a celebration, because Jean Pierre has had some good results from a medical test, and because, well, here I am, their American friend, in Toulouse. And besides, it's a beautiful night!

Beatrice and Jean Pierre step out first. They are like a giggly young couple, holding hands. She's wearing a sweet white linen dress tonight, and I have changed into my favorite blue dress. I am wearing my cute flats. Okay, not flats, exactly. They have kitten heels. The problem is, they also have absolutely no friction to them, and so, as I close the door behind me and I step off the curb and into the street, ready to join arms with my friends, arm in arm in arm, I slip.

It just takes that fraction of a second for the pointy tip on my left foot to become completely wedged underneath a large cobblestone. It's stuck. And then, my heel goes down and gets stuck, and in an effort not to fall forward, my ankle snaps this way and then that way.

I crumble to the ground.

At this point, things began unfolding in a kind of cinematic slow motion. I remember hitting my head against the corner of the brick building, and then the next thing I remember is the sound of panicky voices. Beatrice and Jean Pierre were next to me on the street, telling me to try to stay awake. I came in and out of consciousness, and the next thing I heard were the cries of a siren. Before I knew it, I was being hoisted into the back of an ambulance and rushed to the hospital.

And there, in the back of the moving ambulance, the paramedic spoke to me softly in a lilting, reassuring French. Even in the strange blue light, I couldn't help noticing how young and handsome he was. I admit I felt slightly embarrassed when he held up a little pair of scissors and apologized, but he told me he would have to cut off my tights and ruin them in order to look at my ankle. I told him not to worry about my tights, and so he quickly snipped away and removed the fabric. We both looked at my ankle. It was very red and very swollen. He nodded his head and gently placed an ice pack on it. I vaguely remember him taking my temperature and blood pressure, but these details have faded away. And oddly enough, I felt absolutely no pain and when I arrived at the hospital, I was actually smiling. I also assumed that I had just sprained my ankle. No big deal, I thought, I wanted to spend Sunday in bed anyway! A good excuse to take it easy!

In the emergency room, I remembered actually laughing

and joking. I even had Jean Pierre take a photograph of me in the wheelchair.

But now I realize, I was in a state of shock.

Later, after X-rays and examinations and lots of discussion on the condition of my ankle, reality began to set in. I had managed to break both my tibia and fibula, and I would need an orthopedic surgeon to do an operation. Beatrice and I talked about the possibility of the hospital getting the leg stabilized and immediately putting me on a plane, where I could return home to get the needed surgery. But this would involve finding someone to escort me on the plane from Toulouse to London, and then to Boston. There are no direct flights from Toulouse to Boston. My husband was in the field in Australia and impossible to reach. We did manage to send him an e-mail with the news of my accident along with Beatrice's cell phone number. Plus, we were able to call my father to let him know what had happened. But he is in his late eighties and not in any shape to come and rescue me— although he offered to! Finally, there was my daughter and her husband in Baltimore and my good friend Laurie in New York City. Somehow, I still couldn't imagine how this rescue mission would come off.

And then there was also the issue of blood clots—a concern when you're flying with this kind of injury. But there was something else—this feeling that I had just been asked *so, how much to you love France? How far will you go? Do you trust us with your broken ankle? Do you trust us with a knife? Will you let us operate? What say you now, wayward voyager?*

Sorry, I think I got a little Shakespearean there, but you

catch my drift. This was an opportunity to get to know France from a completely new perspective. The universe was asking me a question. Do you want this thing? Do you want to get on this ride called *The Big French Adventure*?

And my answer was an unequivocal, yes! Yes, I do!

Plus, I knew I would write about it, just like Hemingway wrote about the Spanish Civil War. That man sure had a lot of *ooh la la*!

And so, I was admitted to Clinique Ambroise Paré, where I met with Dr. Delannes. Beatrice knows him and said he was an excellent orthopedic surgeon. Before I could worry too much about it, I was in a hospital room with an intravenous tube in my arm and being prepped for surgery. Dr. Delannes would need to open up my leg in order to realign the bones and then insert a metal plate and six screws in order to hold my ankle together.

And just as the anesthesia was taking hold of me, Beatrice's cell phone rang. It was my husband calling from Australia. I honestly don't remember anything about this conversation. All I remember really is this feeling of joy that we finally got to speak to one another and then a kind of surrender to destiny and a feeling that all would be well in the world, and a certain happiness that I would get to stay and rest at a French hospital, but that my husband would come and get me and bring me home. I felt happy and lucky and then I drifted in and out of consciousness.

I am being wheeled into a huge, brightly lit operating theatre, and there's Dr. Delannes, along with some pretty nurses all dressed in crisp white. They whisper to me in French, but I don't know what they are saying. Nobody speaks English. And my French is floating away from me, and I seem to have forgotten every single word I ever learned. And then, I am out.

In my altered state, I dream that I am taking the train from Toulouse to Valence D'Agen where my friends Cheryl and Jon greet me. We drive slowly over the Garronne River, to the little village of Auvillar, where we pass the church of St. Pierre at the top of the hill. And then coming down the hill, I see pilgrims on the route of St. James Compostela.

My dream shifts to the village. I am talking to my French friend Jo at her restaurant, Le Petit Palais. Jo is wearing a black silk dress with a brilliant green scarf. In the light, it turns blue. And then green again and then blue. She tells me that an English friend bought it for her in Lyon and that Lyon is famous for their silk. I make a note in my little moleskin notebook to visit Lyon and find out about the silk, but then suddenly the scene switches and I am in the caves at Peche Merle. There are a big bunch of us artists and writers on a VCCA/Auvillar fellowship, and I am wearing my slippery kitten shoes into the cave. Amy, a writer, says *we're spelunking in cute shoes*! I want to tell my dream self that this is not a good idea, but it is impossible to speak, and in a flash I am transported to a dinner party in the middle of a field of sunflowers. The beautiful and talented poet Lucy Anderton is sitting beside me. She is very pregnant and she is telling me that a good French hostess will spend ten minutes talking to the guest on her right and then turn and talk to the guest on her left for ten minutes. And then she turns from me and tells the artists and the writers at the table that they should do the same.

Someone lifts a glass of red wine and makes the toast. *A vos amours.* To your loves. We all clink glasses and laugh,

but then suddenly I am alone in the field. It is late in the
season now and the sunflowers have turned black.They stand
in stiff little rows with their heads bowed. I am sad about
this and I think I must come back to the south when they
are in full bloom. I must come back when they are bursting
with color.

Blue. Everything in my dream is blue. I am wearing my
blue feather boa and I find myself at the Bleu de Pastel de
Lectoure, a museum on the history of the woad plant and
in the making of all things blue. I am with my group from
Auvillar, listening as Madame Curator stands before an enormous vat of blue dye and holds an unremarkable-looking
green leaf. *This is the woad leaf!* she announces, and suddenly she appears larger than life. She is wearing a blue
artist's smock and she puts on a feather boa just like mine.
In fact, now everyone in our group is wearing a blue feather
boa!

But I cannot stop staring at Madame. She stands and walks
with her shoulders back, and there is a sense of great dignity; this is when I begin to see that this little woad plant
gives her strength. And then Madame Curator tells us how
the Moors introduced the woad plant to France. The leaves
were crushed and made into a paste, and in the fifteenth century, before ammonia was available, men were paid to drink
a lot of beer and stand outside of taverns so that their urine
could be collected in buckets to be used in the blue dye industry. At this, there are a few giggles in the group, and one
of the artists whispers, *nice work, if you can get it!*

Madame ignores our reaction and continues in all seriousness, telling us that the men in the Middle Ages had two
job choices—to be a soldier and die or drink beer to make
the blue dye.

And then, I feel the softness of my blue feather boa. I am being tickled. Who is tickling me? What is happening here? And this is when I wake up.

French Lessons

Never, ever, ever wear slippery shoes with kitten heels while spelunking—that is, exploring caves. However, it's okay to wear slippery shoes with kitten heels on cobblestones. Yes, you could slip and fall and break your ankle. But you know what? While you might take all the precautions in the world so that something untoward never happens to you, something untoward will still happen. This is the nature of life. And French women certainly know this.

No matter how much emotional insurance we take out, there will always be those events that catch us unaware. The key to ooh la la *is not keeping the unexpected at bay, but it's recognizing the unexpected as an opportunity. Another way of putting this is to make lemonade out of lemons. But it's more than that. When you leave room in your life for the unpredictable, you can embrace it as an invitation to a grand adventure. Don't be afraid, but rather say* bonjour *to the whimsies of life. This is* ooh la la.

!!!

CHAPTER SIXTEEN

～

You Are an Artist

My style is my signature.

—SUZANNE BELPERRON (when asked why she
doesn't sign her jewelry designs)

BONJOUR, MADAME!

I open my eyes to find myself in a hospital bed. In this moment, I have no idea where I am or for that matter, whether I am still dreaming or awake. I close my eyes and go back to sleep.

The next thing I know, a pretty young nurse is opening the shades to my room. And then another one wheels in a tray with a breakfast of a fresh baguette and steaming hot coffee on it. And then, yet another nurse asks me if it's okay for her to lift the bed up and rearrange the pillows. It seems my room is filled with pretty French nurses in crisp white who want to help me. But this is not a dream.

This is the French rest cure!

Actually, it's just the French hospital.

Bonjour, indeed!

A couple of days pass. My husband calls me every day on the hospital landline. He will be coming to get me in a week. He asked if it would first be all right if he visited his daughter who lives in Sydney, Australia, and I said, yes, because after all, I really have no pressing engagements and no place to go.

I spend my day daydreaming and staring out the window at the beautiful clouds overlooking the outskirts of Toulouse.

And now, I'm actually beginning to feel as if this is my new home. My old life before this slowly but surely fades away and I embrace my new life—which is confined to the parameters of this little hospital room.

I make friends with all the nurses and I create little routines and diversions to keep my mind busy. I record the day's schedule in my little moleskin notebook. I take photographs of my leg. It's now kept lifted up off the bed in a brand-new white cast encased in a white fishnet stocking with a seam running up the back. Honestly, it's downright chic. Oh, and then there's the French hospital food! Delicious! For breakfast, I am given a mini baguette, butter, jam, and a cup of *café au lait*. Lunch is the biggest meal of the day with a main course, a cheese course, salad, and dessert course. Oh, and one day they served pâté. Yes, incredible! And delicious. Dinner is lighter and always includes some vegetable soup or broth. I am definitely on the French diet. There are no snacks in between meals—except chamomile tea at ten o'clock, but that's it. No wine. Although when John and Cheryl from Auvillar visit me, John asks if I want him to sneak some in. I say, no, I don't think that's a good idea. After all, I am on a lot of painkillers, including morphine for the first couple of days. That would probably explain those dreams.

No one here speaks English and my French language skills are definitely improving—especially when it comes to medical terms. I've now memorized the French words for *operate, bone, temperature, cast, bandage, blood pressure*, and the all-important *pain*. I know that *montez* means I'd like my bed moved up and *descendez* means I'd like it down so I can sleep. I've learned that a normal temperature is thirty-seven centimeters. A shot is called a *piqûre*. I get one of these every evening.

Fanny and Anne Laure are my favorite nurses. They are so good to me and so sweet. Anne Laure tells me about her husband who works for Airbus and how they have a one-year-old daughter named Lily. She says she wants to learn more English, so we switch off—sometimes speaking in French and sometimes speaking in English.

One day, Anne Laure comes into my room with a tiny circular saw. She places my leg on top of a surgical pad and gets out some instruments. And then she says, *Maintainent, j'ouvre la fenêtre.* I ask her what she means by opening the window.

The window on your cast! she tells me. *I am going to make a little opening so we can see your stitches.*

I nod my head and watch as she takes the teeny circular saw and gently cuts opens two squares—one on each side of my ankle. I actually take a photograph of her doing this. This keeps me from getting too nervous about the close proximity of a saw to the tender flesh of my wounded ankle.

It looks good, she says, and then begins cleaning the incision. She goes on to tell me that she is so excited to meet an American and that she will actually be moving to America for a year!

C'est vrai? (Really?) I ask.

And she says, yes, and that her husband's company, Airbus, is sending them to Kansas for a year.

Kansas!? I ask, laughing a little, because I honestly find it so delightful that this very, very French girl will be transported into the middle of the country—Kansas—home to Dorothy from the *Wizard of Oz*. It seems so delightful to me. *Where in Kansas?* I ask.

Weeesheeetah! She says with great enthusiasm.

Weeesheeetah? I repeat, not quite understanding.

Oui, *Weeesheeetah!*

And then, I get it. Wichita! Wichita, Kansas!

A few more days pass and I am getting better all the time. Beatrice stops by just about every day. And when she returns from a business trip to Paris, she comes back with a little bag of macarons from Lauderee for me. I try to make them last, but it's not easy. Oh, and one is made from rosewater. It's so delicious and fine and kind of like eating a fragrant pink rose that's been dipped in sugar. It's now my new favorite macaron flavor.

Docteur Delannes comes in and visits me every morning to see how the ankle is doing. He's a very handsome man, and I do believe I'm developing a little crush on him, but this could be simply from the fact that he rescued me. Perhaps I am developing one of those doctor-patient complexes. He tells me he speaks no English whatsoever, so this makes him even a little more mysterious, a little more inaccessible.

During the day I read and at night I watch French TV. I do not allow myself TV until after dinner, because I'm really trying to keep up my *ooh la la* and remain present to all the interesting things around me. Still, I must reveal one spicy little tidbit about French TV. They have a miniseries that takes place in a nineteenth-century brothel. It's not as risqué as it might sound, but still—a brothel! Wow. I like to watch it wearing my blue feather boa. In fact, I have gotten into the habit of putting on a nice dress every day, and even putting on my red lipstick. If there's one thing I've learned from the French woman, it is that *ooh la la* is where you find it. And for me, that's in a hospital bed.

One morning, very early, I am awakened by one of the nurses. She tells me she is here to take a blood test. I've been put on Coumadin, an anticoagulant drug, in preparation for my flight home. Coumadin will prevent blood clots. She turns on the light next to my bed. I look at my trusty wristwatch, which I have not taken off since the day of the accident. I should mention that during all these days, I have had no Internet connection or cell phone or even a way to make a phone call out, although I am able to receive phone calls. And so, my little wristwatch, my camera, and my little moleskin notepad have become important touchstones for me. My French is improving, but there are times when I turn my brain off and just listen to the sound of the French speakers without even attempting to figure out what they're saying. It's a dreamy feeling. Almost childlike—hearing sounds with no meaning.

I understand the world from a more instinctual level. I have become more attuned to facial expressions, gesture, and the sounds of the speaking voice. Sounds. I make lots of decisions while I am lying in this hospital bed. I decide that when I get home, I will take up a musical instrument. I will learn to sing. I will spend more time staring out of windows and daydreaming. I will spend less time worrying about my

French grammar and more time memorizing French poems. I will spend less time worrying about my weight and more time dancing.

I will spend more time feeling grateful.

In order not to slip into some kind of hallucinatory state, I write down little notes about what happens during the day and at what time. This way, I will not completely forget who I am or where I am, which feels like a distinct possibility as the days pass by, one after the other.

Bonjour, Madame, the nurse whispers to me.

Bonjour, Madame, I say to her, and then I check my watch. It is not quite six in the morning. From the little window at the foot of my bed, I can see the muted rose-colored light of dawn slowly approaching. The nurse, a pretty woman, somewhere in her thirties or early forties, is dressed in a pristinely white, starched uniform—the kind that our nurses used to wear in the United States maybe thirty or forty years ago—smiles and goes about quietly preparing the little tube and the needle. I am too groggy to tell her that this will not be an easy task. I silently brace myself for the ordeal to come.

Back at home, getting blood work done has always been an ordeal for me. Medical technicians place me in a special chair because I have been known to faint. This is because after being poked and prodded eight or nine times, and then being scolded for having *tiny veins,* or *roly-poly veins*—and once I was actually told I have *deceptive veins*—well, I get a bit agitated. Often, after several false tries, the technician will bring in another technician. She will try the other arm and perhaps on her third or fourth poke, she will find a good vein. But by then I am left with a series of red marks and bruises that will only grow bigger and darker during the coming days.

So you can imagine my delight and surprise when this pretty French nurse felt carefully around the veins on my arm for several moments as if she were a divining rod, and then stopped and chose one. Then, in one seamless motion, this nurse put the needle into the vein and simply drew the blood. *Voilà!*

I look at her incredulously. Tears in my eyes.

Vous êtes une experte. You are an expert, I tell her.

The nurse removes the needle and gently presses a little cotton swab on my arm where the blood was taken. She looks at me and smiles ever so slightly—you know, the way French women will smile at you, giving you just a little peek into their emotional life but still holding a little something back.

Non, she says slyly. *Je suis une artiste.* (I am an artist.)

I have thought about this encounter over and over again. For me, this little early morning conversation has been a grand epiphany, a moment of illumination in my quest to understand what makes the French woman so fascinating. And I believe in this moment, in this French hospital—I had discovered an important answer to my search. This young nurse defined for me the essential secret to the French woman's approach to life, and her wellspring for *ooh la la.*

This idea of approaching life as an artist may seem obvious to some, but it took me a long time to really understand what this meant. I had to go on my own very circuitous journey, interviewing and intellectualizing my discoveries. I had to exhaust myself physically and emotionally before my heart was open to the simple truth.

* * *

I wake up in the middle of the night. It is pouring rain outside. I suddenly feel so sick. My head is pounding. I call for the nurse. She whispers to me that she will get some medicine. And then when she comes back I tell her I think the rain is giving me a sinus headache. She says no, it's *le vent d'automne*.

The autumn winds. And then she goes on to tell me that these winds come to Toulouse every year around October and they whip up all sorts of things—crazy dreams and bad headaches. Women are more likely to go into labor during this time of year. I stare into her face for a moment and I have this feeling that I have encountered a witch. Or Joan of Arc or the Wizard of Oz.

Reality is a land that is slowly shifting away from me and I am standing on an iceberg in the middle of the ocean, and all I know is, it's been nine days here in the hospital in Toulouse and I want to go home.

I click my red boots together three times and whisper, *there's no place like home. There's no place like home. There's no place like home.*

French Lessons

I remember something Micheline said to me in Paris. She's the gal who helped me choose the blue feather boa. She said, "We French, we like to throw a flower on everything." And now, I understand.

If the French were to "brand" their culture and were forced to come up with a mission statement, I think it would be this: to be artful. *I might even add,* to always be artful. *And this applies to every aspect of their lives— whether we are talking about food or fashion or conversation or their love life or professional life. It applies to the simplest and most complicated gesture. And you can see this artfulness when you meet a sophisticated Parisian, as well as the country girl living in a little village in Valence D'Agen.*

Even when a French woman is cleaning out her bathroom, she does it with dignity and grace. For a French woman it is more important to be artful than to be beautiful. This makes sense, because if you think about it, if you are truly artful, you have the ability and the gift to make everything beautiful!

You are an artist.

So, consider this—whether you work in a hospital or bake bread for a living or live in the country or the city or have never even thought much about Art—you are still an artist. You create your own life. And every day, you have an opportunity to take this piece of human clay and mold it into something that is fine and elegant and pleasing. You get to decide what is beautiful, what looks good on you, and exactly how you will go about letting your own light shine. You are the lead in your own Broadway production. You are the painter as well as the model. You are the singer, who performs her own song and dances to her own tune. You are the costume designer, the set designer, the producer, and the director.

And you are absolutely the star of this grand extravaganza called life.

!!!

CHAPTER SEVENTEEN

❦

Now, Voyager

We travel, some of us forever, to seek other states, other
  lives, other souls.

—ANAÏS NIN

I OPEN MY EYES to the rose-colored light of dawn, yawn slightly,
and then drift back into a half sleep. Someone comes into
my room and opens up the window, and a warm autumn
breeze floats into the room. Next, I inhale the aroma of fresh
coffee and a few minutes later, I sit up to find a tray before
me. There is a little bowl of *café au lait*, a baguette, butter,
and two tiny jars of jam. Strawberry and orange marmalade.

"Bonjour," the lady in white whispers softly, fluffing my
pillow before tiptoeing out of my room.

And just imagine—all it took was a broken ankle to get
me to slow down and appreciate the simple joys of breakfast.

At home, I would often skip breakfast. Yes, I have coffee—
lots and lots of coffee, while I peck away at my laptop. No,
not writing something brilliant and wonderful and important. In fact, working very hard at avoiding writing. I am

checking my e-mails! Oh, and in between that, I check my Amazon numbers. And then I read the newspaper before I go back to e-mails and then Facebook—that is, until I find a funny video featuring a kitten and a dolphin cuddling. My husband leaves for work and then suddenly, I realize it's noon and I still haven't had breakfast! By now, I am starving and so I quickly make a bowl of oatmeal with raisins and then eat it up while reading the paper.

And during all this, I never glance out our window—which happens to look out onto Waquoit Bay on Cape Cod. We live in the sort of beachy place that people dream of visiting one day. It's really pretty and people spend lots of money just to find a summer rental. And you know, French people come here during the summer months as tourists!

But I have not truly appreciated this beauty that is in my own backyard.

So, you can see that it was nothing short of a miracle that here in the French hospital, I have actually learned to stop and stare out the window and to truly appreciate my break-fast. And now, I realize I love breakfast! And I love it so much, in fact, that I slow down and I take my time. Yes, and I love dabbing a bit of butter on my baguette, along with a little strawberry jam. Ooh, and I love hot coffee!

And you know what? I don't feel guilty about the butter and bread and jam, because I know for a fact that there will be no food until lunchtime.

And now, just as I am at the point of learning my lesson, it is time for me to go home.

And indeed, I am going home today. At last. My husband, Bill, is here! He is surprised to see that I'm in such bad shape. Apparently, I underplayed the seriousness of the situation. And I suppose I did. I am a fiercely independent woman and

I do not like to be dependent on people. And yet, here I am, completely dependent. The world has certainly decided I have a few things yet to learn. Bill has bought new plane tickets that will take us from Toulouse to London and then to Boston. He arranged for a town car to meet us at the airport and take us directly to the doctor in Falmouth. Oh, and the plane tickets are for first class.

Hey, this is one way to get to fly in first class!

But seriously, I will have to fly with my leg elevated the entire way and so I need a roomy seat. I am forbidden to put any pressure on my leg. I absolutely cannot touch the ground with my left leg, not even for a second. This will be the case for another six weeks. I am given French crutches, which go under the elbows, not the underarms. During the past nine days I have not walked any farther than from my bed to the bathroom and back again.

And now here I am, with Bill pushing me in a wheelchair into the Toulouse airport. We are praying we can get out of the country. There's a national transportation strike that just started in Paris. Beatrice and Jean Pierre joke that there are three ways to arrange for a longer stay in France—a national strike, marrying a French man, or arranging to have your ankle broken. Well, I got two out of three!

We say our *au revoirs* (good-byes) and Bill wheels me over to security. At first, the officials will not let me through. I do have a huge cast on my leg, after all, and who knows what sorts of things I might be hiding inside of it. Perhaps a metal plate and six screws!? Bill holds up the X-ray pictures and *voila*! The French are very impressed by my bravery, my *je ne sais quoi*, my *ooh la la*—and they wave me through with a cheer of *Bonne chance, Madame!*

We are on a British Airways flight from Toulouse to Paris and I will admit it—I am really thrilled to hear the English accents. Heck, I'm just thrilled to hear English! My native tongue.

America, I'm coming home to you!

We have a very entertaining flight assistant in first class. He is very funny in a particularly English way and wants to know if I fell skiing. *No,* I say, *I fell while walking.* And then he laughs, because this does seem like a rather crazy thing. And at this moment, it does to me, too.

Finally, we reach London. And here's the rub. This plane does not go right up to the gate at Heathrow, but rather there are stairs on the outside of the plane onto the tarmac and from there, a bus. Oh, and it's raining and windy out there. I process this. The tarmac! A bus! Stairs!? At this point, the idea of negotiating stairs feels as if someone has suggested I hop down the Rocky Mountains on a pogo stick. *C'est impossible!* (Impossible!)

There is an alternative—the elevated platform that is mechanically lifted to reach the other side of the plane's door—the side where the food carts are wheeled out, along with people in wheelchairs. That would be for me and an elderly gentleman from Germany.

The door opens; the platform is ready. Outside the air is crisp and it's really raining now. In fact, a huge clap of thunder resounds as I am pushed and wheeled out of the plane with a thump and a bump and told to wait a moment. The wind whips up and a blast of cold air hits my face. I look at Bill and he looks at me. And I grab his hand and whisper, *I love you.*

And then suddenly, we are dropping down. The British Airways flight attendant, who is operating the lift, smiles at me sweetly. And knowing that I am more than a little scared, he says, *Oh, luv, just close your eyes and pretend you're at Disneyland!*

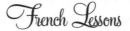

French Lessons

I brought a lot of things home with me—and not just a metal plate in my ankle with six screws—but a pair of red boots, a blue feather boa, a new perfume, and a little brown bottle of Tonique Sexuel.

But more than this, I brought home a new love and appreciation for my husband, the knowledge that I could depend on him when the going got rough. This rescue mission was just the beginning for us. It's a story for another day, but I would like to say that I had a most wonderful convalescence thanks to Bill, his fabulous cooking, and his generosity.

Oh, and I did take home the secret to ooh la la. *And the secret is actually quite simple—it's this: open your heart, feel the love that's all around you, and have the courage to be your own unique self.*

This is the French woman's secret to ooh la la—*she has given herself complete permission to be her unique self. She has completely aligned her outer self with her inner self. This allows for her sense of confidence and mystery. This is what makes her beautiful—whether she is a little overweight or has a slightly crooked nose or is a woman of a certain age. This is* ooh la la.

And for you, this, this ooh la la, *this unique self—well, she's been there all along for you, just waiting for you to claim her. You don't have to go to France and break your ankle, but you might consider staring out the window at clouds, looking at life as an artist, choosing your special color, relaxing and pampering yourself, buying a new perfume, and finding out what your great-great-great-grandmother was like. All these things will bring you close to your truest self.*

So begin your own journey now and say bonjour *to your* ooh la la*!*

!!!

French Women Answer Our Most Pressing Questions

Frédérique

What is your favorite fragrance, and why?

The first perfume I wore was Cabochard from Grès (*cabochard* means "undisciplined"), and I think my grandmother offered it to me when I was sixteen or seventeen years old (what a symbol!).

I've had several favorite fragrances in my life, depending on my age and what was going on in my life. Recently my favorite one was the Eau de toilette Chance, from Chanel. One good French friend of mine—working for Chanel in the USA—offered me this perfume as I was starting a new professional project (in 2009). I liked the fragrance and I needed the chance to succeed, so this perfume became like a talisman.

A few weeks ago, Pierre and I were in an airport and I

tried an Eau de toilette from Guerlain called Idylle. I had a kind of "love at first sight" for it because of the fragrance (like a bunch of flowers, but also something very sensual, I don't know what). Pierre liked it very much, too, and bought it for me. The perfume is also a way to remember the kind of love at first sight (or second sight!) that I felt for Pierre.

From time to time, depending on the circumstances, I will also adapt the perfume. For example, I will choose Shalimar from Guerlain for a Parisian dinner (something very "chic") or on the contrary something very light (I like fragrances from Calvin Klein) when the weather is very hot outside or when I'm in a hurry!

Twenty years ago, I also wore Eternity for Men, from Calvin Klein, to remember a man and my impossible love story with him.

We all adore the French femme d'un certain âge. What do you think is the secret to her elegance, beauty, and style?

These women comfort me over my fear of old age. In a world that glorifies youth, thinness, these women are totally uninhibited and feel good "in their skin" (is that an expression that you also use in the USA?). They take care of themselves, are pretty, and are eager to seduce (themselves and other people). They are positive; they continue to make plans. They are educated and many of them are interested in social issues, so it is always exciting to have a discussion with them. They saw French society change over the years and have an angle of view, a hindsight (is that the right word?) that young people cannot have. So it is always interesting to talk with them because they have ideas to convey; there is always a lot to learn from them. They are witnesses of the past without being nostalgic for a bygone age. They tried to keep the best of the past but at the same time to adapt to changes in society, which I think proves their modernity as well as their wisdom.

They refuse to be locked into one role: many of them have grandchildren but refuse to be available at all times to look after them. They have time as they are retired, but their agenda is full and they don't want to be relegated to the role of nanny, even if they like that role from time to time. However, they are usually generous, giving time to those who need help, through associations for example. They are cheerful and like to have fun, never refusing an opportunity to go out.

They often know well their city or region and always have interesting activities to offer to their friends or family. With them, you never get bored. They continue to love life though they have already done so much along the way and have experienced difficulties, sometimes dramas. The difficulties of life have not knocked them down but instead have given them the ability to enjoy every moment of life, an awareness that we don't always have when we are younger.

They are mysterious because they are probably hiding doubts or adventures they lived: which one of them can say that she never fell in love with another man after she got married or that she never thought about leaving everything to follow a stranger? We must not forget that these women often got married in the fifties or the sixties and that at this time, in France, religion and morality were still very important.

About the special relationship I have with my aunt—it is not uncommon in your family to have a person who is not your mother or father but who is a guide, a model, because he or she meets your vision of life. I spent my childhood alone with my mother, a woman broken by her divorce, who had little interest in my games and dreams.

When I was spending time with my Aunt Odile, I knew I would live an experience as light as a soap bubble. I wanted these moments to last forever. My aunt used to take me regularly with her son and other children (we were usually six children), to the cinema to watch a cartoon, or to the funfair. What was great was to see that she had a lot of fun as well. She was a child among children, but then at the end of the day she would become a mother for her son and a wife to her husband. Her ability to adapt to circumstances still fascinates me. I think this is an essential key to love and be loved in life. I admire her courage, as she took in her life's difficult decisions, which have not always been easily accepted by family members. She is for me a model of freedom because nothing and nobody can dictate what is good or bad for her; she follows her instinct and does not refrain from making difficult choices. She does not judge others and can hear everything; she can keep secrets and provide advice on sensitive issues.

I also admire her willingness to learn, as she comes from a modest family where people work a lot but where there is little time for reading or visiting a cultural exhibition. Odile is interested in many subjects, be it literature, art, nature, social studies. She seeks to understand, learn, and to be open to new emotions. It is a path that I saw her take over the years and I'm trying to take it myself because I think it is a key to personal fulfillment.

Please tell me your top beauty secret; for example, one French woman told me that she believes in ending her shower with an icy cold rinse. Do you have any simple tips on beauty?

Removing makeup before bed, drink water, moisturize. I started in my teenage years, so pay attention. I went to a dermatologist once. Didn't have big acne. I have friends who go for facials. I like to pamper myself (when you have the hot water in a bowl and cover your head).

French women are famous for Le No Makeup look, but still we know that this look involves some makeup. What do you see as the essential ingredients to this look?

Mascara is the one thing. Personally, I do this because I have thin, blond lashes and I notice among my friends, they're not into foundation, yes, they would apply it, not every day. But blush—terra cotta shade. Pinky or bronze powder. Lipstick or lipgloss. In the eyes, very subtle. Minimum. Next step, a little bit of foundation, eye pencil, barely eye shadow. Eyebrows and nails are not as important in France as the United States. Nails are big in the US. In the US it was out of the question I could go without my manicure.

In the cosmetic industry in France, people aren't going to judge you. Same with hair. I have a good friend who's a makeup artist here and he's always in Paris where his boyfriend is, and he's noticed that women are more sophisticated in North America. He tells me, *you French women, what's with your hair? You don't take care of yourself. You don't brush your hair.*

This is true; a lot of women in Paris want to be ready in five minutes. In France, hairdressers are careful to take into consideration the geometry of your face.

Do you ever have that guilty feeling? What brings it on and how do you get rid of it?

I'm not sure; I think we do the same things as American girls. I remember I was thirty years old and we were at my friend's place. It was the typical two girls getting together to chitchat, or maybe it was a way to get over work issues or boyfriend problems. We had this bag of candies and we ate the entire pack, and by suppertime, we said, *oh, my God, I don't feel well.* I remember my belly felt bad. But we just laughed about it and when we see these candies now, we laugh. They're called Dragibus. They're kind of like jelly beans. We felt more stupid about the fact that we were like kids because we didn't know when to stop.

We all adore the French femme d'un certain âge. What do you think is the secret to her elegance, beauty, and style?

The difference is in style and how you choose your fabrics. Unfortunately, all this is disappearing and there's definitely a standardized look in fashion. I'm hopeful that it's not going to be totally over. There are always new designers and new styles. There's Net-A-Porter in the US.

Tell me about your hairdresser.

I always go to the same woman. I've seen women come into her store with a picture of an actress and say they want to look like the actress. But their hair is completely different. But did you know? French women are wearing hair products made in the US more than in France, because hair is so important in the US. We love John Frieda, which is now available in France. Revlon products weren't always available—only in salons, but now French women are buying them. For nails, OPI, the nail polish.

What do you like to bring back from the US that you can't get in France?

I love Raisinettes . . . not available in France!

Isabelle

Please tell me your top beauty secret. Do you have any simple tips on beauty?

A good night's sleep (going to bed early from time to time, in the dark, avoiding noises or avoiding doing something too exciting before)!! It makes the skin looks rested, refreshed, smooth, and glowy.

French women are famous for Le No Makeup look, but still we know that this look involves some makeup. What do you see as the essential ingredients to this look?

I don't wear makeup on my skin, apart from concealer under my eyes to hide dark circles (if any), and some eye lash stuff, and shadows on my eyelids.

To stay healthy, we know it's important to drink lots of water, but do you have any other suggestions like this?

Do some sport and/or relaxation. Protect skin from sun, sleep well and enough, have at least one moment of pleasure for yourself during the day, enjoy every little moment: this is when you glow. Give love to those around you; that's what makes you glow and be attractive. Cultivate positiveness.

When you visit the USA what beauty products or clothes do you look for to bring back to France?

Some beauty brands are quite famous and probably cheaper in the USA: Estée Lauder, Clinique, and Maybelline (called Gemey in France).

I might also buy some American jeans.

What is your favorite fragrance, and why?

My favorite fragrance is from Chanel: Coco Mademoiselle (see the ad with Keira Knightley). It is so refined and feminine, and deep. I feel feminine and attractive when I wear it and it's from Chanel, so of course it adds up to the feeling of "being important" (it's psychological).

Have you ever said no to buying a dress or jeans or skirt or bag, and why?

To say no to what?? I say no to myself if I really don't need an extra bag/jeans/skirt. I can resist buying.

If you've gained a few kilos, what do you do to take them off?

I do running one hour at least once a week. I stop eating junk food, especially *viennoiseries* (croissants and *pains au chocolat*, which contains a lot of cooked butter). I stop munching, I eat more fruits and vegetables, I have regular mealtimes, I have a balanced diet. I drink a lot of water. I don't eat too much for dinner. I am careful on wine and beer.

How do you keep your home free of clutter?

Once in a while (every two years or every year), I do a big cleaning, going through every room and drawer/wardrobe/cupboard, and getting rid of what is not nice/not useful/not used for two years/not making me feel happy, and I throw/give/sell/recycle. Then every day or week, I go through the clutter and tidy up, so it looks nice and neat. I do housework once a week briefly, and bigger once a month.

Do you ever have that guilty feeling? What brings it on and how do you get rid of it?

Guilt about what?

We all adore the French femme d'un certain âge. What do you think is the secret to her elegance, beauty, and style?

Her education, especially from her mother. The old-fashioned style (elegant, smart, discreet). The self-confidence, the will to remain young in her head, happy and attractive, no matter the age.

Please tell me about your Secret Garden. What do you keep there?

In my Secret Garden as you say, I have my sofa, a good book, a hot tea (well . . . plus chocolate biscuits!!), and *silence*. Or sometimes it can be nature plus silence plus all senses open.

Who are your closest friends, and why?

One is my Irish friend Pat; she is very wise, intuitive, spiritual, generous, loving, caring, never judging, and fun. There is so much love in her voice that I can confide in her and it soothes me every time. I have some other few good French friends. I confide less in them (not my deepest emotions and thoughts), but yet they can be supportive, cheering me up, listening, and encouraging. I met Pat whilst I was living and working in Ireland in 1997. She is thirty years more than me, so sixty-eight this year. I think it is her nature to be wise. She has done a lot of work on herself, she is a healer in body harmony, she meditates. And she went through some rough stuff in life.

Anything else you'd like to add? Is there something you'd like to tell American women to help them feel more "French"?

I am very un-at-ease when I read "feel more French." I think it is a horrible thing to say, because they won't be able to change their nationality, it is their heritage. American women have to be proud to be American; it is not healthy to want to become French, to become someone else.

Sylvie

What are your favorite fragrances, and why?

For fall and winter I like Dior Addict from Christian Dior. It's a woman perfume, but a boyfriend of mine was wearing it and it fitted him super well. When I discovered it on him, I decided to wear it.

For summer, I like Cool Water from Davidoff. My mum offered it to me ten years ago and I keep buying it. Last summer I wanted to take a break from it so I bought another one—Jeanne from Lanvin. I chose it with the help of a salesperson at Sephora.

Fran

Please tell me your top beauty secret and any simple tips you'd like to share.

Going for a nice haircut gives a feeling of regeneration, with a good scalp massage.

French women are famous for Le No Makeup look, but still we know that look involves some makeup. What do you see as the essential ingredient to this look?

A little blush is just enough for me.

To stay, healthy, we know it's important to drink lots of water, but do you have any other suggestions?

The other main thing is to move—sport, gymnastics, yoga.

What are the top three things you keep in your Secret Garden?

A book, a record, a piece of art.

Have you ever said no to buying a dress or jeans or a skirt or bag, and why?

I don't like buying clothes.

If you've gained a few kilos, what do you do to take them off?

Sports and gymnastics and being careful with food.

How do you keep your home free of clutter?

I clear up often.

We all adore the femme d'un certain âge. What do you think is the secret to her elegance, beauty, and style?

She takes care of herself and then forgets about it. Other things are more important in her life. She does not want to be appreciated for only her looks.

Anything else you'd like to add? Is there something you'd like to tell American women to help them feel more "French"?

Visit other countries. Learn other languages. Be curious.

$\mathcal{F}inale$

In order to be irreplaceable one must always be different.

—COCO CHANEL

OOH LA LA can come from anywhere. You don't have to travel to France, like I did. It just so happened that this is where I found my *ooh la la*. For you, it might mean simply opening the front door and walking down your own street. You can find beauty in the most unexpected places. Look out at your backyard. Stare at the clouds. Daydream.

This is particularly important.

And finally, you will want to participate in this theater of life. Walk down the street, wearing your signature braids or your favorite fragrance or your green blouse or that blue feather boa. Give yourself permission to be completely yourself. This is how *ooh la la* works. It begins with one woman in one town, wearing something beautiful, unique, and perhaps artistic. This "something" could be as simple as a wool hat she bought at an artisan fair, but this woman with the hat—she is sending out the silent message to the next woman—*be yourself.* And then, this next woman goes home, and takes out that favorite dress she had shoved away in the back of her closet. She cleans it, brings it to the tailor, and then she wears this dress around town. She gets compliments, and she feels the love, and she blossoms. And the more she wears this dress, the more it becomes iconic. And the more the dress becomes iconic, the more the woman becomes iconic.

And she gives other women inspiration to be iconic. To find their *ooh la la.*

In the sea of faces that look exactly the same, with the same smooth foreheads, and the same plumped-up lips, and the same hairstyle, wearing the same outfits and the same shoes—the woman who dares to be the artist and creator of her own unique self is a revolutionary and she has the power to change the world.

Yes, imagine a world where all the women decide they will be completely their own non-air-brushed, beautiful selves. That is *ooh la la*, and it's available at this very moment to you. Just look into your heart.

Acknowledgments

I thank my husband, Bill, for all those months of caring for me, for the delicious dinners brought to me on trays, and for his incredible patience and abiding love.

I thank the good people at the Clinique Ambrose Paré for their wonderful care.

I thank my Dad for all his support and wisdom. I thank my daughter for her creative inspiration. And I thank all my friends who encouraged me, in particular, Minter Krotzer, Jessica Lee, Deborah Krainin, Elizabeth Gold, Nancy Flavin, Deborah Davis, Anne MacAulay, Stephanie Hoffer, Beverly Aker, Julianna McCorkle (assistant extraordinaire!), Tess Link, and Laurie Graff. Oh, and thank you to Jan Elliot for teaching me to play French songs on the concertina, Kelly Johnson for the Zumba lessons and merci beaucoup to the Zumba girls for all the joie de vivre.

Much of this writing was done during fellowships with the Virginia Center for the Arts (one in Virginia and another in Auvillar, France) and I thank them for the time, the space, and the quiet to write. I could not have written this book without the generous French women and American women living in France who opened their doors to me. A big American thank-you goes out to Marjorie Van Halteren, Sylvie Gourlet, Tania Fovart, Beatrice Le Nir, Cheryl Fortier, Josie Mermet, Micheline Tanguy, Sylvia Benito, Heather Stimmler-Hall, Patricia Gellenter, Peter Havas and Coco, Vanessa Gerold, Frédérique Duviqnacq, Odile and the femmes of Rouen, Madame Cadolle, and Isabelle Avril.

I am particularly grateful to the amazing Paula Martin, my creativity and spiritual life coach. She held my hand when I had truly lost my way. I also want to thank my beautiful and brilliant French tutor, Marceline Colton, for all her patience and kindness and inspiration.

I thank my wonderful editor at Kensington, Audrey LaFehr; my brilliant agent, Irene Goodman; and my lovely publicist, Vida Engstand.

Finally, I am so very appreciative of all my sister-(and fellow)-Francophiles and the writers who share my passion for all things French. You've inspired me so much. A big *merci beaucoup* goes out to my readers all over the world, who've written to me and shared their stories and secrets with me. I am moved beyond words. This book is for you.